Praise for *Your Strong, Sexy Pregnancy*

"Practicing prenatal yoga with Desi helped me to maintain my strength and kept my body toned throughout my pregnancy. I worked throughout my pregnancy, so it was very important to me to keep up my fitness and to stay in great shape. My labor was only two hours and I absolutely attribute this to my prenatal yoga. Desi's classes kept me strong right up to the days before I gave birth."

Maxine Bahns, actress, athlete, and mom of two

"Pre- and postnatal movement classes with Desi introduced me to cross-training for pregnancy, labor and delivery, and being a mom. Combining yoga, traditional strength exercises, and a little bit of cardio helped me to feel strong and prepared for labor and delivery. Participating in Desi's class every week completely aided in my healing, both mentally and physically. I don't know what I would have done without her teachings when I became a new mother."

Sandra Kawahito of Mamai, wellness center owner and mom of four

"Trust yourself and know that you have all the answers within. Nobody knows what's right for your child more than you. If something feels right, follow it. If something feels off, follow it. Vibes don't lie. Desi embodies this way of living. She is a wonderful guide for teaching you how to let go of the outside well-meaning voices telling you what you should and should not do, and find a deep sense of center so that you can hear the wisdom of your own inner guidance so you can live more from your truth."

Lori Bregman, doula, healer, and author of The Mindful Mom-to-Be

When I took my first prenatal yoga class with Desi, she had us put a hand on our belly and a hand on our heart and I instantly started to cry. She connected me to my pregnancy in such a special way and helped me stay strong and flexible at the same time. Her class was a safe haven.

Erin Torpey, actress and mom of two

"Desi's approach to safe, effective prenatal yoga with gentle focus on keeping core muscles strong for quicker recovery, along with her calm, confident demeanor is perfect for any mom-to-be!"

Linda Shelton, former fitness editor, Fit Pregnancy magazine

"Prenatal yoga and fitness can benefit women in their third trimester for many reasons, including stretches and strengthening activities that aid in preparation for labor and delivery. As the founder of Bebe PT (or Women's Health Physical Therapy Clinic), I share many clients with Desi. Women experience various physiological changes during their last trimester, many of which can be addressed with specific yoga stretches and poses to help prepare the body for labor and delivery. Desi understands the pregnant body and recognizes when someone needs additional care such as physical therapy or chiropractic interventions. Our shared clients rave about Desi as she is not just a wonderful yoga instructor but so much more to her clients. Her vast knowledge and infectious personality are truly inspiring and I feel honored to be able to work with her and her clients."

Martina Fogt, MPT, CAPP-OB, *specialist in perinatal care, pelvic floor and bowel and bladder dysfunction*

"As a mom, giving birth was the most amazing experience ever. I never thought my body had that much strength and power. In a moment when I was more than exhausted, my body knew exactly what to do. I will never forget the endless joy and love that followed holding my baby for the first time in my arms. As an ob/gyn it is the biggest honor and joy being able to observe and accompany the patients' transition from pregnancy to becoming a mom. Thanks to Desi and her prenatal yoga class I learned to focus on my body, to trust and believe in its strength and power, and to keep on breathing calmly in the biggest pain. Thank you, Desi! I can't put it into words how much you helped us."

Dr. Conny Fendler, OB/GYN

"It is important for a woman to get her doctor's clearance after labor and delivery before she dives back into exercise. Starting with a mindful, gentle yoga practice is a great way to ease back into exercise while your body is establishing a new normal. Desi provides a gentle reentry into exercise for new moms."

Dr. Betty Lee, OB/GYN

"The benefits of Mommy & Me yoga extend far beyond the hour-long class. Yoga with your baby establishes a lifelong pattern for new moms to exercise and care for themselves. Studies show that when mothers exercise, their children tend to be healthier and do better in school. So, when parents ask me what they can do to improve their children's health and well-being I tell them, "Have a daily exercise routine for yourself. Lead by example. Your child will learn discipline and self-care, which is called modeling behavior." It's good for you and good for your child! It's the proverbial win-win."

Lisa Stern, MD, *Tenth Street Pediatrics, Santa Monica, CA*

"I didn't just learn about prenatal and postnatal care in medical school, I made it a priority during my pregnancies and beyond. My youngest child is nearly two years old and I continue to heal, to change, to find the best ways for me to embody the "fit mom" persona I aim to be in order to inspire other moms. Thank you, my fitness guru, Desi Bartlett."

Natiya Guin, ND

"The importance of self-care for moms cannot be emphasized enough. When we neglect our self-care, everything in our life suffers, from our health and mood to relationships. Desi's classes provide moms with a space for mindful reflection and allow moms to focus on strengthening their bodies and prioritizing their own wellness."

Noelle Claudat Fletcher, LMFT

"Lots of our patients speak highly of their prenatal yoga and how it helps them get and stay physically, spiritually, and emotionally healthy through and after pregnancy, but Desi's clients and students rave about her classes and frequently call her work life changing. I had the pleasure of interviewing Desi on the Informed Pregnancy Podcast and was able to experience her magic firsthand. Good fitness professionals can prescribe the right workouts and show you how to do them properly, but Desi's passion makes you want to do them, helps you enjoy doing them, and gives you the strength to follow through long term. Just talking to Desi about fitness has already been transformative for me."

Dr. Elliot Berlin, DC, *founder of Berlin Wellness Group*

Your Strong Sexy Pregnancy

A Yoga and Fitness Plan

Desi Bartlett

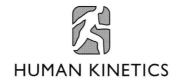

HUMAN KINETICS

Library of Congress Cataloging-in-Publication Data

Names: Bartlett, Desi, author.
Title: Your strong, sexy pregnancy : a yoga and fitness plan / Desi Bartlett,
  MS, CPT, E-RYT200, RPYT, YACEP.
Description: Champaign : Human Kinetics, [2020] | Includes bibliographical
  references.
Identifiers: LCCN 2018058995 (print) | LCCN 2019001558 (ebook) | ISBN
  9781492587538 (epub) | ISBN 9781492569817 (PDF) | ISBN 9781492569800
  (print)
Subjects: LCSH: Yoga. | Exercise for pregnant women.
Classification: LCC RA781.7 (ebook) | LCC RA781.7 .B377 2020 (print) | DDC
  618.2/44--dc23
LC record available at https://lccn.loc.gov/2018058995

ISBN: 978-1-4925-6980-0 (print)

This publication is written and published to provide accurate and authoritative information relevant to the subject matter presented. It is published and sold with the understanding that the author and publisher are not engaged in rendering legal, medical, or other professional services by reason of their authorship or publication of this work. If medical or other expert assistance is required, the services of a competent professional person should be sought.

The web addresses cited in this text were current as of November 2018, unless otherwise noted.

Senior Acquisitions Editor: Michelle Maloney; **Developmental Editor:** Laura Pulliam; **Senior Managing Editor:** Amy Stahl; **Copyeditor:** Rodelinde Albrecht; **Permissions Manager:** Martha Gullo; **Graphic Designer:** Dawn Sills; **Cover Designer:** Keri Evans; **Cover Design Associate:** Susan Rothermel Allen; **Photographs (cover and interior):** Natiya Guin, NMD, M. Ed/©Desi Bartlett; **Photo Production Manager:** Jason Allen; **Senior Art Manager:** Kelly Hendren; **Illustrations:** © Human Kinetics; **Printer:** Versa Press

Human Kinetics books are available at special discounts for bulk purchase. Special editions or book excerpts can also be created to specification. For details, contact the Special Sales Manager at Human Kinetics.

Printed in the United States of America   10 9 8 7 6 5 4 3 2 1

The paper in this book is certified under a sustainable forestry program.

Human Kinetics
P.O. Box 5076
Champaign, IL 61825-5076
Website: www.HumanKinetics.com

In the United States, email info@hkusa.com or call 800-747-4457.
In Canada, email info@hkcanada.com.
In the United Kingdom/Europe, email hk@hkeurope.com.

For information about Human Kinetics' coverage in other areas of the world,
please visit our website: **www.HumanKinetics.com**   E7364

Tell us what you think!
Human Kinetics would love to hear what we
can do to improve the customer experience.
Use this QR code to take our brief survey.

To all mothers everywhere. The light in me recognizes and bows to the light in each of you and in each of your children.

Contents

PART I   Plan for a Strong Pregnancy

1 Strong Is the New Skinny   3

- Live fit from the inside out
- Learn the secret of a strong core
- Become strong and sexy throughout your pregnancy

2 3 + 1 Total Body Fitness   9

- Use various forms of movement to create your total body fitness program
- Combine yoga, resistance training, cardio, and nutrition for a healthy pregnancy

3 Mama Knows Best   21

- Connect with your body and become fully present in your pregnancy
- Use meditation to bond with your baby
- Cultivate an awareness of your own and your baby's needs

PART II   Prepare for Birth and Beyond

4 First Trimester: Increase Endurance   33

- Learn how exercise can carry you through your pregnancy
- Use yoga, meditation, and cross-training to fight off fatigue

5 Second Trimester: Build Strength   75

- Get strong for the rest of your pregnancy
- Find a rhythm and establish a regular exercise routine

PART III   Practices for Recovery and Results

Contents

Pose and Exercise Finder

Pose	First trimester	Second trimester	Third trimester	Recovery	Page number
90-90 Stretch				X	268
Alternating Reverse Lunge				X	241
Arm-Only Pointer Dog Pose				X	157
Bent-Knee Fallout				X	154
Bent-Over One-Arm Row		X			89
Boat Pose With Baby				X	190
Bow Pose				X	266
Bridge Pose				X	155
Burpee				X	240
Butterfly Pose	X				65
Chair Pose Into Boat Pose				X	264
Chaturanga Pose				X	244
Child's Pose	X				59
Clock Squat		X			84
Crescent Lunge	X				62
Dancing Warrior		X			86
Deep Relaxation Pose	X				66
Donkey Kick				X	263
Down Dog Pose	X				44
Down Dog Pose Into Stacked Hip Variation				X	162
Easy Pose	X				41
Easy Twist With Baby				X	194

> continued

> continued

Pose	First trimester	Second trimester	Third trimester	Recovery	Page number
Firedancer Squat				X	258
Fish Pose				X	196
Fish Pose on Foam Roller				X	239
Flying Baby				X	191
Foam Roller for the Glutes				X	237
Foam Roller for the IT Band				X	238
Foam Roller for the Latissimus Dorsi				X	236
Foam Roller for the Spine				X	166
Forearm Plank Pose				X	161
Forearm Side Plank Pose				X	213
Fortune-Teller			X		117
Garland Pose	X				63
Gate Pose	X				61
Goddess Pose		X			88
Half Forward Fold	X				46
Half Sun Salutation	X				48
Half Sun Salutation With Backbend				X	163
Heart-Opening Pose	X				64
Heart-Opening Stretch on Stability Ball			X		116
Heel Squeeze				X	159
Hero Pose				X	195
Hip Circle			X		105
Isometric Abdominal Contraction				X	153
IT Band Twist	X				57
Jumping Lunge				X	260
Kiss-the-Baby Chaturanga Pose				X	186
Kneeling Hip Abduction			X		114
Kneeling Sun Salutation With Baby				X	192

Pose	First trimester	Second trimester	Third trimester	Recovery	Page number
Lateral Stretch on Stability Ball				X	165
Legs-up-the-Wall Pose			X		118
Locust Pose				X	222
Lower Back and Hip Stretch		X			92
Lunge With Baby				X	188
Modified Chaturanga Pose	X				51
Modified Handstand				X	242
Modified Side Plank Pose				X	267
Mommy-and-Me Sun Salutation A				X	184
Mountain Pose	X				45
Pigeon Pose	X				56
Pike Pose on Stability Ball				X	214
Pilates Roll-Down				X	219
Pilates Roll-Down With Oblique Twist				X	220
Plank Pose	X				50
Pointer Dog Pose	X				43
Pointer Dog Pose With Abdominal Flexion				X	221
Prone Bent-Knee Lift				X	158
Prone Leg Lift on Stability Ball				X	215
Puppy Pose		X			83
Running Man				X	261
Seated and Supported Wide-Legged Forward Fold			X		108
Seated Extended Side Angle Pose			X		112
Seated Goddess Pose			X		110
Seated Head-to-Knee Pose (Open Variation)			X		109
Seated Pelvic Roll			X		115
Seated Side-to-Side Rock			X		111

> continued

> continued

Pose	First trimester	Second trimester	Third trimester	Recovery	Page number
Seated Thread-the-Needle Pose			X		107
Seated Twist				X	217
Shoulder Press With Baby				X	189
Sphinx Pose				X	223
Squat				X	257
Squat Jump				X	259
Squat With Baby				X	187
Standing Hip Abduction		X			90
Standing Lateral Stretch			X		106
Standing Push-Up		X			91
Straight Leg Crunch With Hip Raise				X	243
Straight-Leg Raise				X	160
Sufi Roll				X	218
Sun Salutation A	X				52
Sun Salutation B		X			80
Supine Hand-to-Big-Toe Pose				X	167
Supine Hand-to-Big-Toe Pose With Twist				X	168
Supine Stability Ball Pass				X	216
Supported Backbend on Stability Ball				X	164
Tree Pose	X				55
Unicorn and Rainbow Pose	X				42
Unilateral Isometric Hip Flexion				X	156
Up Dog Pose	X				54
Upright Hero Pose With Hip Lift	X				60
Upward-Facing Table Pose	X				58
Wall Squat			X		113
Warrior 3 Pose With Hands on Wall				X	262

Foreword

I was first introduced to Desi more than twenty years ago by our meditation teacher who just knew we would hit it off and become instant friends. We discovered that we both had a deep passion for working with pregnant and new moms, health, healing, and empowering women. Throughout the years, we studied all kinds of healing modalities together. Her work with yoga and fitness blended beautifully with mine as a doula and coach. We've supported thousands of women throughout their transformation into motherhood.

Years later, Desi became pregnant and I got to be her doula with both of her sons. Her births were quick and, even though she birthed some big, beautiful babies, she pushed them out with ease and confidence. Desi had found the profound joy and wonder in the entire experience of becoming a mother, and she shared that expertise with pregnant and new moms through classes, DVDs, and private client sessions, helping them to feel deeply connected to their babies and to their own bodies.

I was so blown away by the difference in the birth experience of women who worked with Desi versus the ones who didn't. These women were all strong and empowered in birth, and I noticed that even their labors were faster. Needless to say, after seeing this with my own eyes, I began to encourage all of my clients to connect with Desi. I, too, wanted to learn her secrets, so I signed up for her prenatal yoga teacher training. It was fantastic, and I learned so many things that I use with my clients for birth prep and delivery.

Desi walks her talk. She brings magic to all the mamas who get to learn from her. She is passionate, gifted, and intuitive beyond words. I am so excited for this book and for all the moms-to-be and new mamas in the world who get to learn from Desi's wisdom. I know firsthand that what she teaches really works!

Lori Bregman, celebrity doula, author of *MAMASTE*
and *The Mindful Mom-to-Be*, and cofounder
of Seedlyfe superfoods for all stages of womanhood

Preface

In 2008, I became pregnant with my older son, Cruz. For a fitness professional, preparation usually means dieting down for video and photo shoots. But I knew that preparing for motherhood would not involve shrinking in any way. Instead, it was the time to expand my strength, both physically and emotionally. Those two types of strength are tightly interrelated, especially for pregnant women: Labor and delivery (and motherhood itself!) require both bodily and mental fortitude, so building physical strength to prepare for the very real challenges of labor and delivery (L&D) also builds feelings of confidence and capability.

I sang to my belly every day, exercised, meditated, you name it. I was open to the process of labor and delivery being something that could be empowering. In the middle of the night on September 8, I suddenly woke up and realized the TV was on. Britney Spears was in her lost years, and she was onstage at the VMAs. As I looked up and thought, "Poor Britney . . . I wish I could invite her over for dinner," my water broke. (Aren't the details that we remember about the birth of our children funny?) My husband called the doctor, who basically said, "Stay home, have a glass of wine, and relax for a little while, then head to the hospital when the contractions get closer together." But my husband was too excited and couldn't wait for all that, so off to the hospital we went about 45 minutes later.

A few hours after we arrived at Cedars-Sinai Medical Center in Los Angeles, I was given Pitocin. I had recently seen Ricki Lake's movie *The Business of Being Born* and was afraid that Pitocin would lead to both an epidural and a Cesarean section. If you are not familiar with Pitocin, it brings on a stronger contraction to get the labor and delivery process moving along. The stronger contraction means more pain. More pain usually leads to an epidural and often, the movie asserts, to a C-section because many babies cannot tolerate the Pitocin, which can lead to fetal distress. Needless to say, I was scared.

I am forever grateful that I chose to have a doula present for the birth of my baby. My doula and I decided together that an epidural was the way to go after the Pitocin. I was in a lot of pain, and wanted to take the edge off. Unfortunately, someone forgot to turn off my epidural, or at least to turn it down, and I was completely numb from the waist down. When it was time to push, I could not feel anything, not even much pressure in bearing down. I decided to call on my muscle memory to recall what it felt like to train my

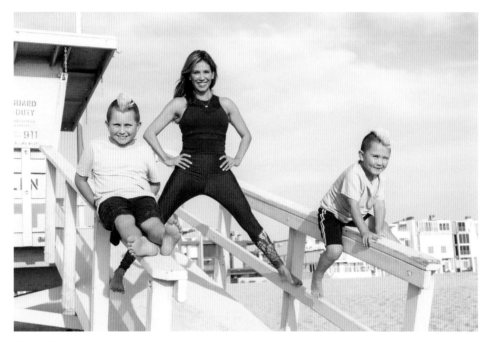

Cruz, Nico Rocket, and me.

pelvic floor and deep core muscles, and how to bear down. In my mind I envisioned these muscles working together to help my baby move easily into the world. I could imagine my transverse abdominis (TVA) drawing in and my pelvic floor pushing down, all while supported by the back muscles. Fifteen minutes later, Cruz Roman Bartlett entered the world reaching for his mama.

With my second son, things were a little bit different. It's true what they say: No two pregnancies are the same, even for the same woman. This time around, I had not gained as much weight because I was very active with Cruz around. I felt strong and ready, and I knew a bit more about what to expect. What I did not expect is that they told me that if I didn't induce at 39 weeks, I would have a 10.5-pound baby. So induce we did. Again I was given Pitocin, and again I chose to have an epidural. My water broke on its own, and this time I made a point of asking for a lower-dose epidural so that I could feel what I was doing. I am happy to share that Nico Rocket Bartlett arrived on December 31, 2013, in just three pushes!

Mothers Into Living Fit: The Beginning

When I was pregnant with my first son, Cruz, I would daydream about bringing him to mommy-and-me yoga classes. At my six-week postpartum check-in with my ob/gyn, she told me that I was clear to exercise, and I was so excited to bring Cruz to a yoga class. About a week later, we went to mommy-and-me yoga at a local studio. The first 20 minutes of class, my son slept in the car seat. When he woke up, he was hungry, and it took about 20 minutes to feed him. After he ate, he wanted to be held, so I cradled him in my arms and we enjoyed some sweet bonding time while the beautiful yoga music played in the background. After class the instructor said, "I'm sorry that your son did not let you practice yoga." At that moment, I heard brakes screeching in my head and felt my Mama Bear energy rise up. I was thinking, "My child is wonderful and his actions are age appropriate, and I was having a nice experience until you said that!" Instead of expressing that to the teacher, I said, "Thanks for class," and quickly left. It was at that moment I knew there was a better way.

The very next day, I watched clips from every mommy-and-me yoga video that I could find. I also attended classes at a different studio, and I started to see what this format could be. The potential for practice to be a sweet, lovely bonding experience with your baby was there. I quickly learned that most babies like to be held most of the time, and that many of the yoga poses could be practiced with baby in your arms. Each day I would set up a warm fuzzy blanket at the front of my yoga mat, and my son would lie in the cozy space that I created for him. Each time I passed through the vinyasa sequence (plank, chaturanga, up dog, down dog), I would give him kisses or make noises like a horse whinnying, or the giddy-up clicking sound to make a horse run faster. Cruz loved the sounds and the belly kisses, and he especially loved when I would hold him in the standing poses. It was a process of trial and error to find the right grip for him to be comfortable and secure, and for my wrists to be in a neutral position. Together, we created sequences based on what he enjoyed and what felt good to my body.

That was the beginning of Mothers Into Living Fit mommy-and-me yoga. Cruz and I brought the format to studios and mommy centers around the city, and together we continued to cultivate a practice full of singing, dancing, yoga, and joy. Fast-forward to today, and my almost-10-year-old son assists in class when he has a day off from school. Watching him check in on moms and babies, and help make babies giggle, and play peekaboo with adorable toddlers makes my heart swell with joy and with pride. He taught me how to teach this format with the valuable feedback that he provided as a baby. Now he is helping as an assistant teacher. This has been valuable to me on so many levels. The two most important lessons that I have learned from this experience are (1) mommy is baby's first role model of health and wellness and (2) baby is (very much) a teacher to mommy.

Acknowledgments

Thank you to everyone who has contributed to Mothers Into Living Fit and *Your Strong, Sexy Pregnancy*.

Special thanks to the following people:

Jeff Bartlett, my husband, best friend, and partner in this life path of raising sons

Cruz Bartlett and Rocket Bartlett for making me a mommy and setting my career on the path of service to families; you light up my world and I love you

Michelle Maloney for helping to shape this project from the very beginning

Laura Pulliam for editing the book and creating continuity

Mike Soenen for believing in me and being a great friend

Alicia Silverstone for being a beautiful example of natural motherhood

Felicia Tomasko for supporting me as a writer, teacher, and friend

Natiya Guin, my photographer, model, contributor, and friend; you are amazing

Lori Bregman for being my doula, bestie, and all-around source of support for making dreams come true

Michele Meiche for guiding my path and contributing a meditation to help guide all moms

Dr. Thomas Sattler for teaching me biomechanics and kinesiology; you are the best exercise physiology teacher on the planet

Kali Sampson Alexander for contributing your yoga nidra skills and divine rest

Shannan Yorton Penna for believing in Mothers Into Living Fit from the very beginning and for your yummy recipes

Jennifer Wells McCauley for supporting me and nerding out on biomechanics for moms; I adore and appreciate you so much

Victoria Davis Dodge for your unsurpassed vegan culinary skills

Liz Vaccariello for giving me my first video job with *Better Belly Yoga* and for sticking with me as I now work with deep core work for moms

Acknowledgments

Jane Fryer for showing me what being a true yoga teacher is all about

Travis Eliot for helping to make this dream happen

Theresa Sauter for showing me the true meaning of mom strength

Kimberly Mampe for sharing your story and Gia Perrone for being my *comadre*

Yael Cohen Braun for your support and enthusiasm

Kate Hudson for being such a beautiful expression of motherhood and strength and inspiring me while I was writing about being a strong and sexy pregnant mama

All of the beautiful moms who have attended my classes, watched my videos, and read my blogs for the last 10 years—it is my honor to serve you, and you inspire me daily

Plan for a Strong Pregnancy

STRONG IS THE NEW SKINNY

3 + 1 TOTAL BODY FITNESS

MAMA KNOWS BEST

Strong Is the New Skinny

Strength from the inside out: that's the goal of the Mothers Into Living Fit workout. Moms cultivate strength on all levels—physical, mental, and emotional—that we can call on for support throughout the journey of pregnancy and into new motherhood. What's at the heart of this strength? Your abs, which we call your *core*. Whether this is your first pregnancy or your fifth, a powerful core is crucial for carrying the weight of the baby and ensuring that mama can move with ease and minimal pain. And no, I'm not necessarily talking about rocking a shredded six-pack until month nine. A very tiny portion of the population is able to maintain the visible cuts of musculature in the abdomen during pregnancy, but those women are so overglorified by some (aka unrealistic expectations) and so vilified by others ("She cares more about her abs than the baby!") that it's really confusing to figure out what a healthy pregnancy is supposed to look like.

In my view, a true Mother Into Living Fit mama is created from the inside out. It's about her self-confidence and her ability to prioritize her health and happiness—and that of her little ones—over what other people might think about her. Whether her belly is soft around the edges or highlighted by muscular lines is not the issue. What's important is how she feels: strong and sexy in every way.

Learn About Your Inner Core

How do we get to the point where we want to take a sexy selfie, or at least be OK with the mother-in-law paparazzi following us around after we give birth? This takes us right back to the core! The core—aka the stabilizing muscles of the trunk—is made up of two main layers of muscles. One is the six-pack muscles everyone thinks of when they think of great abs. Those are the rectus abdominis muscles. But the real secret to a strong core is underneath: the transversus abdominis, or TVA for short. The TVA muscle is shaped like a corset and wraps around your abdomen. Fit mothers know that the TVA provides a strong foundation for posture, gives stability and compression to the internal organs, and supports the weight of the pregnancy.

The TVA muscles also link up with an incredibly important muscle group called the pelvic floor (see figure 1.1). The pelvic floor is a hammocklike layer of muscle and connective tissue that supports organs such as the bladder, intestines, and uterus and, when you're expecting, provides safety and support for your growing baby. The muscles are closely connected to the TVA, and keeping them strong and supple may also make labor, delivery, and recovery easier (not to mention reducing your risk for incontinence issues).

Remember, whatever your favorite workout may be, the rule for fitness during pregnancy is this: If you did not do it before pregnancy, now is not the time to start. Here's what you *can* start doing: training your TVA and lower back muscles. *But wait! I didn't train these muscles before pregnancy, and didn't you just say not to do anything I didn't do before?* The truth is, you absolutely did (and still do!) train these muscles, all the time; each time you walk, lift something, or simply stand up, you engage the core and the erector spinae (lower back muscles). They are required for many, many everyday movements. And now is the time to target these muscles in a more challenging way that will help empower you throughout your pregnancy.

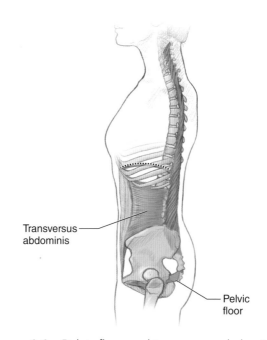

Transversus abdominis

Pelvic floor

Figure 1.1   Pelvic floor and transversus abdominis.

As you progress in your pregnancy, a healthy core will absolutely help you with your posture. Good posture is often linked to higher feelings of self-esteem. When you stand tall like a queen or in a power pose like Wonder Woman, research shows that fatigue is reduced and there is an improvement in positivity of mood. So it's not just about looking good; it's about feeling good from the inside out.

One of the greatest gifts you can give your baby is your good mood. According to Thomas Verney, founder of the Association for Prenatal and Perinatal Psychology and Health (APPPAH), "Positive maternal emotions have been shown to advance the health of the unborn child." He continues, "Thoughts which infuse the developing baby with a sense of happiness or calm can set the stage for a balanced, happy, and serene disposition throughout life." This is not to say that we have to be happy every minute of every day. Life happens: traffic, politics, work stress, you name it. But positive thoughts are a form of nourishment, and just as we can benefit from having a predominantly healthy diet, we can benefit from predominantly positive thoughts. When there are moments of stress (which we all have), try to slow down, breathe, and send your baby love at that very moment.

Become a Fit Mom

Why is the core so important for a strong and sexy body throughout pregnancy? And is training the core while pregnant even *safe*? We're learning more than ever about prenatal fitness from a scientific perspective, partly because it wasn't until the 1980s that anyone even bothered to do studies on the subject. One pioneer was Dr. James F. Clapp III, who spent years analyzing the physical capacity of the pregnant body. He reported on many of his research findings in his book *Exercising Through Your Pregnancy,* in which he notes, "The combination of exercise and pregnancy has a greater training effect than that produced by training alone." Translation: We have the potential for *amazing* results if we continue to exercise while pregnant. There's power in that beautiful belly.

Fast forward to the 1990s, when we saw the first viral image (before we even used that term) of a seriously sexy pregnant woman: the gorgeous Demi Moore and her unclothed bump on the cover of *Vanity Fair*. Little by little, women—especially celebrities—started to share more about their pregnancies. Now that we are well into the 21st century, everyone from athletes to rock stars has begun to celebrate the bump. From Beyoncé rocking four-inch heels during pregnancy to Gal Gadot filming *Wonder Woman* while pregnant, we now have lots of beautiful and strong role models who show what a fit pregnancy can look like.

OK, but you might be wondering: *Isn't it a celebrity's job to look amazing, whether she's pregnant or not?* That's true, and I can tell you from experience as a Los Angeles–based yoga teacher who works with plenty of big

Mommy Move

Unicorn and Rainbow Pose

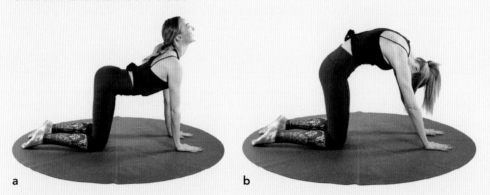

a   b

This move is traditionally called *cat and cow*. During pregnancy, the last thing I wanted was to think of my body as a cow, so I changed the name to Unicorn and Rainbow. Here's how to do this move.

1. Begin on all fours with your hands shoulder width apart and your knees hip width apart. If you need extra padding under your knees, you can place a blanket there for cushion.

2. With your inhalation, take your gaze to the sky as you lift your chest and tailbone and feel the gentle stretch down the length of the front of the body (see figure a).

3. With your exhalation, round your spine and create a rainbow shape around your baby (see figure b). Be careful not to overtuck the tailbone as you round because that could shift the baby inside you.

4. Enjoy several rounds (10 to12) of Unicorn and Rainbow, envisioning your crown rising with the inhalation and an arc of light around your little one on the exhalation.

Information No One Tells You

You Can Be Pregnant and Sexy

Reframing our image of the pregnant body can begin with the language that we use. I encourage moms-to-be in my classes to use terms like *goddess* when talking about themselves and other pregnant women. The ability to carry life in our bodies is nothing short of miraculous, and remembering that a pregnant body is strong and vital is important. Self-confidence and strength are sexy. Others are drawn to these qualities. Sexy does not only mean sexual; it can also mean attractive, confident, and engaging.

Remember that lower back strength is an integral part of core strength. Standing tall like a queen is very different from standing like a person with a backache. In

2010, a study was performed to research the effects of power poses versus yoga poses on the participants' self-esteem. Whereas power poses (e.g., standing with your hands on your hips) can increase interpersonal dominance and power, yoga poses were shown to increase self-esteem. Another reason to enjoy yoga during pregnancy and beyond is that it has been scientifically shown to improve posture and increase self-esteem.

Love-Your-Baby Visualization

Envision Your Belly as a Sanctuary

Take time throughout the day to pause and close your eyes. Enjoy a full, deep, centering breath. Take your attention to the baby inside you and envision your little one within the sanctuary of the space that your body has created just for him or her. In your mind's eye, envision your baby's home as a sacred space. Send your love to your baby, and imagine light within your belly, as though you were shining the light of your love onto your baby's face. With each breath, imagine that light expanding like the rays of the sun at dawn. Continue this feeling of expanding the light with each breath until you sense, see, and feel your entire body as a vessel of light. When you are ready, bring your attention back to the room you are in, and know that you can connect with this feeling of holding light within you at any time you wish by simply closing your eyes and enjoying a deep centering breath. Note: In the romance languages, to give birth is to *give to the light*.

Fun Foods

In the Ayurvedic tradition from India, it is said that root vegetables help us to invite grounding energy. It's thought that when we enjoy foods that grow from deep within the earth, they help us connect to the energy of Mother Earth. Root vegetables include foods like beets, yams, and carrots. These foods also tend to be high in fiber and, as any pregnant woman can tell you, fiber is your friend! With the increase of progesterone during pregnancy, it is common to have days when you are irregular (that's a nice word for constipated). As an added bonus, ginger is commonly recommended by natural health practitioners as a way to help relieve nausea, which is common in the first trimester.

Grounding Smoothie

    1 carrot, scrubbed and chopped
    1 beet, scrubbed and chopped
    1 orange, peeled and segmented
    1/2-inch piece of fresh ginger, grated
    1 cup water
    1 cup ice

Combine ingredients in blender. Blend until smooth.
Yield: *1 serving*

name clients that many celeb moms' motivation to stay in shape is not just for their own health and wellness, but in many cases for their career. And of course they have access to many high-end fitness programs, private chefs, and even surgeons. Some decide to go on a 30-day cleanse after pregnancy, or to have plastic surgery (like those who plan a combination C-section and tummy tuck). It's not my place to judge, but I will tell you that there is another way. The Mothers Into Living Fit program is designed to help you stay strong throughout all the days of your pregnancy, into the delivery room, and beyond. You can feel great in your own body, have the strength to deliver your baby into this world in whatever way you choose (C-section or vaginal, drugs or no drugs, home or hospital), and recover quickly. This sustainable, healthy movement is not a onetime quick fix; it's a lifestyle. And guess what—as you'll read from some of the quotes throughout this book, many celeb moms are embracing strong over skinny, too.

If you're still cringing when I suggest you train during pregnancy, you're not alone. Despite the aforementioned growing evidence that exercise is good both for mom-to-be and for baby, there's still a lot of controversy surrounding the topic. One reason may be that with the rise of the CrossFit movement we're seeing more moms doing workouts that look too extreme compared to what we expect pregnant women to do. CrossFit mom Lea-Ann Ellison inspired lots of nasty online comments when a photo of her crouching down for a heavy dead lift at eight months pregnant made the rounds. Proving the haters wrong, Ellison gave birth to a healthy baby boy and, five months after delivery, weighed *less* than she did before becoming pregnant. But while many moms-to-be swear by it, intense exercise may not be OK for all mamas. That said, a deconditioned body (that's a nice way of saying *out of shape*) isn't optimal for carrying the weight of pregnancy or recovering quickly, either. That's why Mothers Into Living Fit mamas live somewhere in the middle. We are intelligent, discerning women who live an incredibly healthy *balanced* lifestyle.

Years ago, Oprah Winfrey said, "When you know better, you do better." This powerful message has stuck with me. Our pregnancies in this day and age are much different from those of our mothers' generation. Gone are the days of sitting on beanbags and having a cigarette to relax during pregnancy (yes, this was the advice given to my mother!). Thank goodness researchers in our lifetime have taken the time to show us what is safe during pregnancy and what is not. We now know more than ever how to take care of ourselves and of our growing babies.

Yoga, fitness, meditation, a clean diet, and a positive attitude are all elements of a healthy lifestyle. Not only can we look great on the outside standing tall in our strength, we can feel even better on the inside knowing that the baby we carry is benefiting from this positive outlook and lifestyle. Whether you are trying to conceive, are already pregnant, or are a new mom, the Mothers Into Living Fit program can help you stay motivated and inspired. We cultivate power on many levels and we share this with our children.

3 + 1
Total Body Fitness

For many years, I have understood the power of cross-training. Training in more than one way gives us multiple benefits. When I was studying for my master's degree in corporate fitness at the University of Illinois at Chicago, Dr. Thomas Sattler, a member of the National Fitness Hall of Fame Museum & Institute, taught us that there are five main components of physical fitness:

1. *muscular strength* (how much weight you can lift),
2. *muscular endurance* (how many times you can lift that weight),
3. *cardiovascular endurance* (the condition of your cardiovascular system),
4. *flexibility* (your ability to stretch at a given range of motion), and
5. *nutrition* (as it relates to your body fat and body composition).

After many years of working as a personal trainer, I realized that bringing all of these factors together would call for hybrid workouts. Very often I would have my clients start the session with a cardiovascular warm-up, move on to weight training, and conclude with stretching and a little nutritional counsel. As I honed my craft, I found that by adding exercises from many different forms of movement, from boxing to ballet, my clients would see even greater results.

Yoga has been a part of my life from the time I was a child attending services at the Temple of Kriya Yoga in Chicago. The temple featured the symbol of *om* on the wall. One day, as an adult, I was looking at the symbol and realized that it looked like 3 + 1. At that moment, the idea of 3 + 1 Total Body Fitness was born.

3 + 1 represents

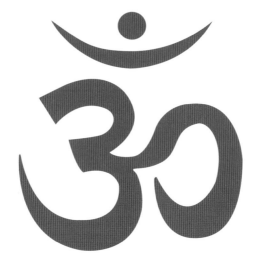

3 (yoga, resistance training, cardiovascular training) + 1 (nutrition).

As someone who grew up with yoga, I found it natural to create the 3 + 1 program with yoga as the foundation. Yoga unites movement and breath; it's a wonderful place for moms to begin on the path to fitness.

Yoga

The Sanskrit word *yoga* means *union*. The union of breath and movement is the most common meaning. Others point to the union of body and mind, and link these words to become *bodymind*. This is how yoga is different from stretching or pure flexibility training; there is a focus on uniting different parts of the self. There is absolutely the idea of stretching the body that helps to improve our flexibility, but that is just one element. We learn from the teachings of the great Indian sage Patanjali that yoga is a rich and varied tradition based on eight principles or, as he called it, the eight limbs of yoga, which are

1. *yamas* (ethical standards, or self-regulating behaviors),
2. *niyamas* (self-discipline, or inner observances),
3. *asanas* (physical postures),
4. *pranayamas* (breathing techniques),
5. *pratyahara* (sense withdrawal, or gaining control over external influences),
6. *dharana* (concentration of the mind),
7. *dhyana* (meditation), and
8. *samadhi* (ecstasy, or the state beyond meditation).

Don't worry; you don't have to burn incense or levitate to practice yoga, nor do you need to memorize the names of the eight limbs of yoga. What is important here is simply to remember that yoga is not just about how deep our Forward Folds are, or how many cool pictures of handstands we can post on Instagram. There is a rich tradition that recognizes that we are more than just our bodies. Our breath is part of our life force, our minds are capable of turning inward to withdraw from outside stimuli, and our ability to concentrate can lift us to deep levels of meditation. So when someone asks you if you are practicing yoga, please know that the yoga sequences that you find in this book are based on the ancient traditions, but with special considerations for the life of a modern mom.

In our modern world, we spend a lot of time leaning forward. Whether we are driving, eating, working on the computer, or gazing lovingly at a baby, our daily habits call for leaning forward so often that the posture muscles are compromised and we look more like we are hunching over than standing tall. This hunching over is called *thoracic kyphosis* and can lead to tremendous tension in the postural muscles. Yoga teaches us how to draw the shoulder blades together with special attention on the breath cycle. This powerful work helps to create new postural and breathing patterns so that you can stand tall like a queen.

During pregnancy, there is an exaggerated curve in the lower back. This swayback posture is normal to the extent that the body needs to compensate for the baby growing in the abdomen, but sometimes it becomes overexaggerated and the anterior tilt of the pelvis causes lower back pain; this is called *lumbar lordosis*. We always have some amount of lordosis and it is important to remember that we are not trying to fix this curve during pregnancy. However, simple exercises that help you to lengthen the tailbone and gently engage your abdominal muscles can help to support the weight of your baby and decrease lower back pain.

An easy way to remember these two types of postural misalignments are to think of a hunchback and a duckwalk. To check out your own posture, set the timer on your phone to take a picture of you from the front, and then another from the side. Look at your feet and notice if they are turned out slightly. Look at your shoulders and notice if there is any rounding forward or hunching. Finally, look to see if your head is reaching forward; ideally your ear, shoulder, and hip should line up one above the other. The practices at the end of chapters 4 to 6 and 8 to 12 will help you achieve a more regal posture so that you stand tall like a queen and not like the hunchback of Notre Dame or Donald Duck.

Resistance Training

According to the American College of Sports Medicine (ACSM), "Resistance training is a form of physical activity that is designed to improve muscular fitness by exercising a muscle or a muscle group against external resistance."

In order for a muscle to get stronger, it has to be challenged. Resistance training allows us to challenge our muscles in a myriad ways using dumbbells, barbells, machines, resistance bands, and other external resistance equipment. It's important to remember that lifting the weight of your own body is also resistance training. If you are at the park with your kids and hanging from the monkey bars, that too is resistance training because you are holding up the weight of your body. Resistance training, also known as weight training, has a long list of benefits. Here are a few. It

- improves bone density,
- increases lean muscle mass,
- strengthens muscles and connective tissue,
- can help alleviate depression,
- decreases your risk of diabetes,
- prevents back pain,
- improves balance, and
- increases body confidence.

If you're a pregnant mom, make sure you are working out in a safe way. If you have never lifted weights before, then having your doctor's clearance before you call a personal trainer is very important. Let me repeat the rule: If you were not participating in the activity before pregnancy, then pregnancy is not the time to begin. But we all need to lift the weight of our own bodies, so please make sure that you have your doctor's clearance for light resistance training. If you do want to add some light weights (in the form of 5- to 8-pound hand-held weights) to prepare for lifting your baby, make sure you are working with a highly skilled personal trainer, preferably one who has pre- and postnatal exercise certification and experience.

If you have trained for many years and feel comfortable in the gym, take the time to familiarize yourself with contraindicated movements (exercises that you should skip for now), many of which are listed in chapter 4. There is a lot of crossover with exercises that are not recommended in weight training while pregnant, and those that are not recommended in the practice of yoga while pregnant. Remember that your belly is a sacred space for your baby, and it is quite literally your baby's home. We never want to lie on the house, crunch the house, or overheat the house. Your little roommate—or, as some mamas say, your wombmate—needs a safe and protected space.

Many yoga postures double as resistance training exercises. The movements are almost identical in many cases, and for our purposes in this book, the resistance training is really designed into the yoga practices, primarily in the form of your own body weight. Exercises like squats, lunges, plank, and bridge are all present in the practice of yoga, and will help to empower you with the strength that you need to help carry the pregnancy in a more comfortable way, as well as to recover faster after baby is born.

Squatting for a Better Booty

Squatting and lunging are my favorite lower body exercises. Lunges, sometimes called split squats, are incredibly effective in helping to increase strength and definition in your legs and your gluteal muscles (glutes). Both of these exercises are portable, meaning that you can do them anywhere, at any time, with no equipment other than your own body weight. In working with thousands of women over the years, I've found that many women, including myself, lose some tone in their derriere during pregnancy. The booty gets a little bigger with the extra weight from pregnancy, but after the baby is born, it can feel as though your bottom fell down. The metaphor I used was that during pregnancy my rear end looked like a plum and after I gave birth it looked like a prune. You might be asking *What helps?* Squatting helped lift and fill out my backside, and it can be done throughout pregnancy and beyond.

You will see squats in almost every form of exercise. Our bodies are designed to bend at the knees and hips. There are many different types of squats: sumo squats (aka pliés), plyometric squats, single leg squats (aka lunges), goblet squats, and the list goes on. Squatting has many benefits, which include strengthening the glutes, the front of the thighs (quadriceps, or quads), the hip extensors (hamstrings), the calves, and the core muscles. In the world of physical therapy, doctors refer to these muscles as the *posterior chain*. It is common for the posterior chain to be somewhat neglected because as a society we have a tendency to sit a lot, and because it's human nature to train the muscles that we can see in the mirror.

Moms benefit from posterior chain training during pregnancy and after baby is born. During pregnancy, there is a shift in the center of gravity, in addition to the weight of the beautiful baby pulling the belly forward. All of this leads to a tense lower back and a weak posterior chain, unless you are training. And then, after baby is born, there is a lot of sitting and holding baby on one hip. Several imbalances can occur between your abs and your lower back as well as between your hip flexors (the largest of which is the psoas) and your hamstrings. Training your glutes correctly can help to correct some of these common muscular imbalances. A few posterior chain exercises that can help balance your muscular strength, and ultimately your posture, are squats, lunges, dead lifts, bridges, and hip extensions.

After baby is born, you can invite your baby into a lot of these exercises; the weight of your baby becomes the resistance that you train with. Typically, most babies weigh somewhere between 5 and 9 pounds and gain a few ounces of body weight each week. In fitness, we learn that in order to avoid strength plateaus our bodies need a little bit more of a challenge every few weeks. Mother Nature has built in a naturally occurring incremental challenge in the form of your baby, who is continuously growing. Each week that you lift your baby (with proper mechanics), you are getting stronger and stronger as you adapt to the increase in baby's body weight.

Evergreen Exercises

Have you ever noticed that almost all fitness magazines look the same? There's always a model doing some form of a lunge, and usually some type of abdominal crunch, too. This is because the exercises that are tried and true are timeless. In the world of marketing, this is called *evergreen*, referring to content that does not change. The same is true for yoga magazines; in almost every publication, you are likely to see a photo of a model meditating and another one of a model in Downward-Facing Dog. After years of purchasing these magazines in search of new movement, I realized that there are a lot of exercises that overlap from one system to another, and are in fact truly evergreen. Here are some examples:

Yoga	Fitness
Chair Pose	squat
Goddess Pose	plié
Crescent Lunge	lunge
Hand-to-Big-Toe Pose	front kick
Chaturanga Pose	triceps push-up
Plank Pose	plank
Forearm Plank Pose	forearm plank
Side Plank Pose	side plank
Boat Pose	pike
Locust Pose	superman

With exercises overlapping, and with so many that look the same from one system of movement to another, you might be wondering *What is the best type of exercise?* The best answer I have ever heard to this question was from my friend and former Miss Olympia competitor Joanne Lee Cornish, who said, "The best type of exercise is the exercise that you *will* do." Finding a form of movement that you enjoy can be just as important as the benefits of that type of movement. Joy will keep you in it for the long haul, and can benefit your body, mind, and spirit. I love yoga and fitness, and see the benefits in both. When a movement does not feel great for one of my clients, I have a separate set of tools that I can draw from. The joy of movement comes in many different formats: yoga, fitness, dance, Pilates, walking, indoor cycling, high-intensity interval training (HIIT), and the list goes on and on. Look for similarities in the various systems of movement. It is usually in the movements that overlap in various systems that you will see the ways that the body is designed to move. Our bodies are clearly designed to squat, stand, bend over, twist, walk, push, and pull.

Cardiovascular Training

The American College of Sports Medicine (ACSM) defines cardiovascular training as "those that are rhythmic, continuous and performed with large muscles of the body.... The goal is to exercise for at least 10 consecutive minutes at a moderate to vigorous intensity level. The talk test is one way to monitor your workout intensity."

Mamas-to-be ask about the safety of all types of cardio, from Zumba to swimming. I can't say it often enough: If you did not do it before pregnancy, now is not the time to start the activity. Many types of cardio are considered safe for pregnancy, including walking, swimming, water aerobics, Latin dance, treadmill, elliptical machines, StairMasters, indoor cycling, and the like. Choose something that makes you feel great while allowing you to keep your heart rate in a moderate zone. If you want to know what the best form of cardio is, my answer is, again, the kind that you *will* do. Choosing something that is enjoyable makes you much more likely to stick with it. As a trainer, it is my goal to help set you up for success.

After baby is born, you can amp up the cardio a little bit, but do so gradually. The first few weeks after you have had a baby are still a delicate time. Take your time rebuilding your cardiovascular endurance by walking with your baby. In a few short months you can consider investing in a jogging stroller and increasing your pace, but it is recommended to start slowly so that you build on a solid foundation.

Investing in a heart rate monitor at this time is a great idea. Monitoring your heart rate during pregnancy can help you make sure that you are working in a zone that is neither too high nor too low. If you choose not to buy a heart rate monitor, you can check your intensity by means of the *talk test*. While you are exercising, do a little bit of talking. The exercise should not be so easy that you can sing nor so hard that you cannot say a few sentences. If you are pregnant, try talking to the baby inside you. These days, so many people have earbuds and Bluetooth that no one thinks you're talking to yourself anymore. You can speak gently to the baby inside and let it know how much you love it.

You might notice that you don't feel as much movement from your baby when you go for a long walk during pregnancy. Please know that this is normal. Your pelvis is like a built-in cradle. With each step forward, you are softly rocking the cradle and soothing your baby. Many babies will take a little snooze while you work out. Something no one tells you is that it is also totally normal for babies to have a dance party in your belly when you are trying to go to sleep. You are not rocking the cradle then, and very often they are active and ready to move. One of my students told me she thought that she was going to give birth to a rock star because her baby would nap during the day and party at night. It is all part of the wild adventure of pregnancy.

After your baby is born, ease yourself back into cardio with walking. Walking with your baby is a sweet way to bond with baby, get some fresh air, and start to walk off some of the baby-weight. It is not necessary to go for very long walks to enjoy the benefits of weight loss. Shorter exercise windows a few times a day can help you to achieve your goals. A morning walk and an evening walk several times a week can help you clear your mind too. Listening to your favorite music, smiling at your baby, and taking in the beauty of nature can be a form of moving mediation and bring you back to a deep sense of center.

In a few months, you will most likely be ready for a greater physical challenge. When you are ready to amp up your cardio, you can pull out that heart

Safe and Sound

Sometimes during pregnancy, our balance is a little bit off. Please take necessary precautions to prevent falling or slipping. Choosing the proper footwear with good traction is a great place to start. When using a treadmill, it is fine to place your hands on the heart rate monitor or even on the sides of the treadmill. If something falls while you are on the treadmill, do not bend over to pick it up (it happens more often than you think). Remember to turn off the machine before you recover the item that fell. Lastly, make sure that the floor or exercise surface that you are using is clean and dry. If there's sweat on the floor of your gym or your yoga studio, it's OK to ask the staff to run a mop over the floor before you exercise. You are not being high maintenance; you are being safe and protecting yourself and your baby.

For those mamas who live in extreme temperatures, please take your cardiovascular activities indoors. Pregnancy and extreme temperatures don't go well together when you are exercising. The pregnant mama's body should never reach a temperature above 100.4 degrees because this can cause damage to the baby's neural tube. At the other end of the spectrum, extreme cold also poses dangers such as frostbite or slipping on ice. If the outside temperature is too cold or too warm, consider joining a gym, investing in a treadmill, or finding a mall walking program in your community.

rate monitor again and start to notice how you need more of a challenge to avoid plateaus. Just as with resistance training, there is an adaptation response with cardio, and you will need to gradually increase the intensity, the duration, or both. The good news is that you will enjoy something called the afterburn. *Afterburn* is the nickname given by exercise physiologists to excess postexercise oxygen consumption (EPOC). Studies show that after we participate in an intense workout, the body continues to burn calories while it slowly returns to homeostasis. This simply means that, just as it took work for your body to run or enjoy a HIIT class, it takes work for your body to come back down to your normal resting state. This makes you what fitness author Covert Bailey used to refer to as a "better butter burner."

Nutrition During Pregnancy

Nourishing our bodies is very different from being on a diet. It is important to remember that what nourishes your body might be very different for your best friend or even for your sibling. Each of us has a unique body chemistry, a unique sense of taste, and—depending on the demands of our day— different caloric needs. Finding balance in a world that promotes extreme diets can be a bit challenging, not to mention that sometimes you simply might not like the food or food group that is being promoted. Nutrition as a component of fitness is more about making sure that your energy needs are met in the form of calories and that the food is not being stored as excess fat that could be detrimental to your health.

Pregnancy is not the time to diet. Your body will naturally have clear and distinct preferences that might be very different from month to month. For example, I found that I could not be in the same room as cooked eggs during pregnancy and felt super nauseous when I smelled them, even though this was a food I enjoyed before pregnancy. On the hand, I craved lemonade all the time. I know the high amounts of sugar that can be in lemonade, but I still found myself reaching for more. I began to suspect that pregnancy cravings represent something deeper, something primal.

In his book *Magical Beginnings, Enchanted Lives*, Deepak Chopra tells how food aversions are a part of our evolution. A cavewoman did not have the resources to ensure that meat or chicken was prepared in ways that would be sure to kill off all bacteria, or that the surfaces used were not cross-contaminated; she simply knew that something smelled gross. This was her biology speaking to her to protect the baby inside. Food aversions are an evolutionary part of protecting our species. When you look at it that way, it is much more interesting than just needing to leave the room because someone prepared a food that is not palatable. You can say to yourself, *Wow, my body is protecting my baby*.

As for cravings, in my experience it is quite common to see moms-to-be reaching for foods from their own childhood; Pop-Tarts, peanut butter and jelly sandwiches, and breakfast cereal with characters on the box are often favorites. There is a psychological component at play here, as well as a craving for carbohydrates. The psychological component has to do with craving foods that were familiar or comforting to us as children. Pregnancy is a huge life event, and craving something that we associate with comfort to ease us through this period of change makes perfect sense. Also, craving carbohydrates makes sense because of the increased energy needs associated with making bones, organs, and a placenta. Making a baby takes work.

Balance is the key to proper nutrition during pregnancy and beyond. From the Western teachings of health and nutrition, we are taught that it is incredibly important to stabilize our blood sugar. Finding the correct balance of carbohydrate, fat, and protein that works for your body can leave you feeling satiated and energized and maintain a healthy body weight and body composition (ratio of fat to lean muscle mass). Make sure that every meal includes

- high-quality carbohydrate (e.g., fruit, vegetables, steel-cut oatmeal, brown rice),
- protein (e.g., tofu, tempeh, lentils for vegans; eggs and lean meats optional for those who are OK with animal sources),
- fat (e.g., avocados, extra virgin olive oil, nuts), and
- water, for the hydration needs of the mother and the placenta.

From the Eastern teachings, we are taught a different view on balance, which is very well defined by researcher Amala Guha at the University of Connecticut's School of Medicine. In her teachings, what is referred to as an Ayurvedic diet "asserts that every root is a medicine so there is no good or bad food and provides a logical approach to designing balanced foods for optimal nutrition by formulating food groups that work in harmony, induce proper digestion, and promote maximum absorption of essential nutrients."

*M*ommy Move

Breathing Into the Corset

We have deep abdominal muscles, the transversus abdominis (TVA), that help support our bodies from the inside out, much like an old-fashioned corset. The TVA is often active without us even thinking about it, much like our heart continues to beat without us needing to think about it. When we focus on these deeper belly muscles, we can start to feel how they work in harmony with the diaphragm and the pelvic floor muscles. We learned about the TVA in chapter 1; it can be helpful to remember that these muscles are located behind the abs.

Here is a detailed exercise to help you feel this harmonious relationship of the inner corset with the structures above and below it.

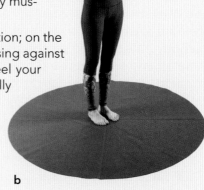

a

b

- Begin in Mountain Pose with your hands on your sides like a corset (see figure a).
- Breathe deeply and feel that, on the inhalation, the entire abdomen expands out to the sides. Feel that your trunk (that's a less sexy word for torso) is filling like a balloon.
- Pause for a moment with the belly completely full of breath.
- Exhale slowly, feeling the deeper belly muscles move in toward the center.
- Your hands can assist you with this action; on the inhalation, feel your belly gently pressing against your hands, and on the exhalation feel your hands gently pressing against your belly (see figure b).
- Enjoy several rounds of this deep awareness in your abdomen so that you can connect to the feeling of the TVA acting much like an inner corset, helping to support your organs.

*I*nformation No One Tells You

The Body's Changing Colors

The abs are made up of a long sheath of muscle that runs from the bottom of the sternum (breastbone) to the pubic bone. The muscle has two halves and meets in the center with powerful connective tissue. On the skin we can see this connection;

it is called the *linea alba* (white line), a whitish line that runs down the belly. Because of the change in hormonal levels, an interesting thing happens during pregnancy: This line can turn a very dark brown; it is then called the *linea nigra* (black line). This change occurs in up to 75 percent of pregnancies and is simply a hyperpigmentation, much like darkened nipples or melasma (mask of pregnancy). This dark line usually disappears a few weeks after delivery. What no one tells you is that if you exfoliate the skin after baby is born, the line will disappear faster. Some moms use alcohol on a cotton ball; others use sugar scrub to help remove dead skin cells. Both methods are effective.

Love-Your-Baby Visualization

Nourishing the Placenta

Close your eyes and envision your baby's back to your belly, with the head pointed down toward your pelvis. Now envision the placenta, a flat organ that helps nourish your baby via the umbilical cord. Invite slow, deep breaths and start to stretch during the length of your inhalation as well as your exhalation by a second or two. Continue to breathe deeply, and imagine that you are drinking in what the yogis call *prana*, which is life force energy. Let each breath bring in prana, oxygen, and light, and now imagine that this beautiful luminous energy is being shared with your baby across the placenta, through the umbilical cord. Instead of eating for two, imagine that you are breathing for two. Each deep breath is a gift to your baby because it helps to release feel-good chemicals in your body, signaling that all is well and you are safe. Share these thoughts with your baby and send your love and blessings to the little one who will be one of the loves of your life.

Fun Foods

Back in the 1980s, it seemed as though every shopping mall in America had an Orange Julius at the food court. Bright orange signs and delicious orange-and-vanilla-flavored shakes were not to be missed when we were shopping with girlfriends. As delicious as these treats are, the high sugar content can spike your blood glucose levels, especially during pregnancy. As we know from the world of physics, what goes up must come down. When our blood sugar spikes, it will eventually crash, leaving us tired and craving more sugar. To get off the wheel of blood sugar spiking and crashing, it is important to add some protein to our sweet treats. Here is a recipe for a yummy, protein-packed version of an orange and vanilla treat.

Healthy Vanilla-Orange Shake

> 1 tablespoon vanilla protein powder (my favorite is Quest)
>
> 1/2 cup freshly squeezed orange juice
>
> 1/2 cup almond milk or coconut milk
>
> 3/4 cup ice
>
> Dash of vanilla extract, to taste

Combine ingredients in blender. Blend until smooth.
Yield: *1 serving*

Ayurvedic teachings assert that the taste of foods, called the *rasa*, can be categorized as

- *sweet* (promotes strength, but in excess can lead to being overweight; e.g., dates, cashews),
- *salty* (maintains electrolyte balance, but in excess can cause water retention; e.g., celery, sea salt),
- *sour* (stimulates digestion, but in excess can lead to heartburn; e.g., lemons, tomatoes),
- *pungent* (improves digestion and can clear sinuses, but in excess produces extreme thirst (e.g., ginger, onions),
- *bitter* (said to help with pancreatic function, but in excess can lead to dizziness; e.g., turmeric, coffee), and
- *astringent* (said to help with nutrient absorption, but in excess can lead to constipation; e.g., parsley, chickpeas).

As a lifelong student of both Eastern and Western teachings, I like to integrate the best of both worlds, look for consistencies in theories, and identify ways the ideas can complement each other. For example, if I have a cold, I use a neti pot (Eastern) and take vitamin C (Western) to get better as quickly as possible. I encourage you to look at both Eastern and Western philosophies on nutrition and notice that the overlapping idea is balance. Finding a balance of foods to support your needs during pregnancy and beyond is a win-win for mom and baby.

Throughout this book, you will find recipes in the Fun Foods section at the end of each chapter. These recipes offer natural remedies for nausea and other ailments common during pregnancy, as well as satisfying the natural cravings for comfort foods in the healthiest way possible. After baby is born, finding a balanced diet helps give you a renewed sense of energy and supports you in nursing (if that is your path); this is also addressed in later chapters. Remember that your needs will change for each trimester and for the time after your baby is born as well. Be gentle with yourself and make choices that allow you to feel balanced and nourished from the inside out.

Yoga, resistance training, cardiovascular training, and proper nutrition are a powerful combination that can allow you to walk tall with strong muscular support, enjoy healthy heart and lung function, and have a healthy ratio of fat to lean muscle tissue. The exercise programs at the end of chapters 4 to 6 and 8 to 12 , along with walking and proper nutrition, will create a solid foundation of strength, flexibility, and cardiovascular endurance, and help to keep your body fat within a healthy range. Take your time adding new exercises and activities. Fitness is not a race; it is a lifestyle that can help you throughout your journey into motherhood.

3

Mama Knows Best

Women have been having babies since the beginning of time. Throughout the centuries, we have evolved in such a way that there are built-in safety systems to protect the baby inside you. Food aversions are an example of your internal safety system. Uncooked meat or eggs might make you nauseous because your body is trying to keep you safe and let you know that is not safe for the baby inside you. The same is true for exercise. If there is a movement that you just don't feel right about, think of this as valuable feedback from your internal safety system. This is also the birth of your new and powerful skill: mother's intuition.

"Mother's intuition is the deep intuitive blood bond a mother can have with her child," says psychiatrist Dr. Judith Orloff, author of *Guide to Intuitive Healing*. "It is a sixth sense mothers have that the child may be in danger or in need." For mothers, having an intuitive bond with your baby is a beautiful experience, and can help guide you in the journey of motherhood. With so many voices chiming in on what we should or should not do, it can be challenging to know which voice is right, and what is the right answer. The truth is that there is often not just one correct answer when it comes to being a mom, because every mom and every baby is unique (even twins). If you are new to the idea of tuning in to your energy system and listening to the feedback of your body, mind, and heart, then cultivating this awareness during pregnancy can help you connect to the energy system of your baby as well.

Connect to Your Inner Energy System

In the practice of yoga, the spine is called the tree of life, and on this metaphorical tree we see a rainbow of energetic centers that the yogis call chakras. The Sanskrit word *chakra* translates to *wheel* or *disk*. There are seven main chakras, each corresponding to a different color and life theme (see figure 3.1). The first three chakras are said to be the chakras of matter (*muladhara*, *swadhisthana*, and *manipura*). This simply means that these first three chakras relate directly to the physical body. The fourth chakra, the heart chakra, is said to be the place where matter (your physical body) connects to your spirit. The upper chakras (*vishuddha*, *ajna*, and *sahasrara*) are said to relate directly to your spirit or soul or essence (whichever word resonates most with you). When you are grounded in the chakras of matter and the physical

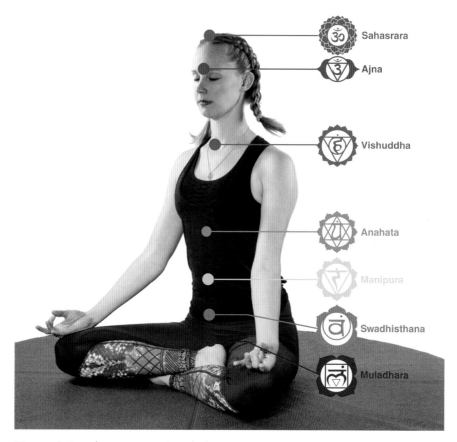

Sahasrara

Ajna

Vishuddha

Anahata

Manipura

Swadhisthana

Muladhara

Figure 3.1 The seven major chakras.

world, there is a feeling of being fully present as a mother. The chakras of spirit allow you to connect to all that is, and to be aware of your connection to the universe and to universal energy. The chakra that connects earth and sky is your heart. It is your heart center, the compassionate heart of a mother and unconditional love that bonds to baby.

When studying the chakras, try to stay playful and open-minded, like a child. Let the idea of the inner rainbow simply be a metaphor for different aspects of yourself. Each aspect has a different theme, and focusing on each one individually brings awareness to any imbalances. It can also bring an awareness of new joys, perhaps like the joy when you first find out you are pregnant. Here is a deeper look into each theme.

First Chakra

The first chakra, or root chakra, is found at the base of the spine and corresponds to our foundation and to our ability to feel grounded, rooted, and fully present in our bodies. This first center also relates to the ability to trust, and is depicted by the color red.

Second Chakra

The second chakra, or sacral chakra, corresponds to our sexuality and creativity. The sacrum is that big, wide bone in your lower back just beneath the waistband of your pants, and has the same root as the word sacred; many people believe this to be a special or sacred part of the body. The second chakra is found at the level of the sex organs and relates to our ability to connect with another person sexually. It is depicted by the color orange.

Third Chakra

The third chakra, or solar plexus chakra, can be found a few inches above the navel; it corresponds to matters of power and self-expression. This is the center that is active when we feel strong in our posture (a strong core depicts confidence), as well as when we have a true belly laugh. This center is depicted by the color yellow.

Fourth Chakra

The fourth chakra, or heart chakra, is found at the level of the heart and is said to be the energy center that connects matter (your body) and your spirit. This center corresponds to matters of love and healing and relates directly to our ability to love and embrace, which is integral to being a mother. This center is depicted by the color green, although it is interesting to note that many pregnant women report experiencing it as pink.

Fifth Chakra

The fifth chakra, or throat chakra, is found at the level of the throat and corresponds to matters of communication and to our ability to fully express our truth. The fifth center is depicted by the color blue and is integral to clarity of speech.

Sixth Chakra

The sixth chakra, or third eye chakra, is found at the level of the forehead and corresponds to our inner vision. When we close our eyes, we see an inner image or picture. This center relates to matters of awareness and to having an expanded vision (beyond what is right in front of our eyes). It is depicted by the color indigo.

Seventh Chakra

The seventh chakra, or crown chakra, is found above the crown of the head. This energy center corresponds to our connection to whatever your name is for something greater than humankind: life, nature, all that is. The crown chakra color is often depicted as violet, although some traditions occasionally depict it as white.

The chakras cannot be seen with the naked eye. If our body is opened during surgery, no one will see a whirling disc of light in our belly. By the same token, even though we cannot locate our personality at one particular point in our body, it is still in there. There are parts of us that we cannot see, but we know that these parts help to make us who we are. The subtle energies that make up the chakras are easier to experience when we are in meditation. When we close our eyes, we can connect to the vision of a certain color or a specific feeling that we experience in a particular part of the body. In our daily life, it can be very easy to sense a particular energy center in relationship to another person that we have strong feelings for or about.

As we interact with individuals, there can be an energetic connection from one of our chakras to that of another person. I know this can sound a little woo-woo or out there, but if you think about someone you love dearly and take a moment to notice where you experience this in your body, you might notice very clear feedback. Perhaps, as with new love, you feel it in your tummy, like the butterflies the first time you talked to your crush on the phone. Perhaps you feel it in your throat, as in wanting to declare your love; think of every song you've ever heard that includes some version of "I can't hold back" or "I've just got to tell you."

These connections from your energy system to another person are called energetic cords. Generally speaking, it is recommended that we not have a lot of energetic cords with others. It is better to keep our own energy system

Body Wisdom

There are many different rules and guidelines regarding exercise during pregnancy. In my opinion, the single most important guideline is if your mind, body, and heart are telling you to stop an exercise, then it is time to stop immediately. Your body holds wisdom and will let you know if an exercise is not right for you. You might feel a little apprehensive about a movement and not necessarily be able to explain why, or you might actually feel some physical discomfort. Even if an exercise is deemed safe during a particular trimester, that does not mean that your body will adapt well to every exercise on the list. You are an individual and your pregnancy is unique; it is important to honor this clear feedback from the body.

There are some occasions when a woman should immediately stop exercising and call her doctor. Here is a list of reasons to cease exercise immediately, according to the American College of Obstetricians and Gynecologists (ACOG):

▌ Bleeding from the vagina

▌ Feeling dizzy or faint

▌ Shortness of breath before starting exercise

▌ Chest pain

▌ Headache

▌ Muscle weakness

▌ Calf pain or swelling

▌ Regular, painful contractions of the uterus

▌ Fluid leaking from the vagina

clear and not always be thinking about, talking about, or daydreaming about another person (good or bad). There is one huge exception to this rule. The energy cord that runs from the heart of the mother to the heart of her baby is a healthy cord. Much as the umbilical cord supplies nourishment for the body, the energetic cord provides emotional and energetic sustenance. Sending love from your heart center to your baby's heart center is a sweet experience for mother and child. By affirming this bond in meditation, you can help to strengthen the emotional bond while your baby is still in your tummy, and when baby is born, you will very easily connect to a mother's intuition.

Connecting With Your Baby in Utero

During my first pregnancy, I spent a lot of time meditating. I would often go for long walks and then sit on the beach to connect to my son's energy. I loved to sit cross-legged in front of the ocean and send love to my little boy. One day, I was feeling a sweet sense of love in my heart and I had the clearest vision of dolphins jumping out of the water. For a moment I was not sure whether I was looking at real dolphins playing in the Pacific Ocean or I was in meditation, seeing dolphins in my mind's eye. Eventually I realized that I was deep in meditation and that it felt as though these dolphins were being sent to me, like when someone sends you a video on your phone. I held that image in my mind but did not think about it again for a few weeks.

About two months later, I was in full-on nesting mode and eager to get the nursery ready. A good friend of mine paints murals and offered to paint one on the nursery wall. She asked me what I would like her to paint, and I knew immediately: dolphins. The dolphins were painted above the changing table, and after my son was born he would always stare at or point to the dolphins. When he was old enough to speak in full sentences, he said, "Thank you for my dolphins, mommy." I knew at that moment that the image I had seen in meditation was a message from my little boy.

I know that life is full and busy for many women. Especially if you already have little ones, taking the time for meditation during a second or third pregnancy can be challenging. Please know that a little goes a long way. The intuitive bonding meditation takes only about five minutes in total, and you can do it anywhere: on the train, in the passenger seat of a car, or in the tub. It does not require a two-hour of window of time to connect to your baby. Once I realized this, I started bringing this meditation into the prenatal yoga classes that I teach in Los Angeles. Each class closes with a short, sweet bonding meditation for mommy and baby.

One day in class, I decided to ask the mamas-to-be if anyone would like to share what they experienced during meditation. The stories were amazing. One mama reported that for months she and her husband had not been able to decide on a name for their baby, but that during meditation she heard her baby's name so clearly that she knew it was meant to be. Another mama shared that she had a very clear vision of the mountains and saw herself and her daughter playing in the mountains. This same mama also shared that in her vision she saw her daughter as about two or three years old. Amazingly, about two years after her daughter was born, they moved from the beach to the mountains. There are many stories like this, and I see them as beautiful examples of the intuitive bond between mother and child.

Take a few minutes each day to connect with your baby. Breathe deeply, and enjoy this sweet time when your baby is still inside you. Send your love and blessings to your little boy or little girl. Talk or sing to your baby. Notice if you feel any flutters or kicks. The baby inside you can feel what you are feeling, and inviting the feeling of love is a gift to both mother and child.

The meditation that follows offers you an opportunity to recognize and foster this energetic connection with your baby.

Begin this meditation seated with your legs crossed in Easy Pose. Close your eyes while bringing one hand to your heart and one hand to your baby. Slow your thoughts. Slow your breath. Imagine that each breath is a little slower and deeper than the last one. Gently allow your attention to drift to your heart center. The heart center is located at the center of the chest. In Sanskrit, it is called anahata chakra. Anahata means unstruck, referring to the poetic idea that the organ of the heart is constantly beating, like a drum that does not need anyone to strike it from the outside for it to continue its steady rhythm. Notice if you can sense, see, or feel a particular energy in your heart space.

As you connect to your heart space, invite the feelings of love and compassion. Connect to a feeling of expansion with each breath. Every time you inhale, imagine the feeling of love growing in the heart space, like the rays of the sun, and let this love radiate out with warmth and light. Imagine a beautiful silver cord of light originating in your heart center, softly extending and connecting to your baby's heart center. Envision this cord of light like an old-fashioned telephone cord and use it to send messages of love to your baby. Perhaps you simply say or think the words I love you or I am so excited to be your mommy. Whatever feels natural to you is the right thing to say. Sit with these feelings of love emanating from you to your baby for at least a minute.

After a minute or so, allow yourself to be the receiver of the communication. Notice if you are having any thoughts or feelings that don't seem to have originated in your own consciousness. Many healers from around the world believe that babies in their mama's tummy communicate in images. Notice if there are any images flashing in your mind's eye that might be a message from your baby. Do you see his little face at four years old smiling up at you? Or perhaps her voice whispering in your ear what she would like her name to be? Try not to dismiss any feedback.

Also, remember that you are your baby's entire universe. You have their favorite voice, their favorite smell, and they already love you. Let yourself feel the power of your baby's love for you, and know that out of all of the millions of possibilities in the universe, you and your baby have come together.

If it were possible to take a picture of a feeling, imagine yourself now taking a picture of this beautiful bond of love between you and your baby. Let your baby know that this loving bond that you share is special to you, and that you will cherish this feeling of love as you move through the rest of your day. Close your meditation by envisioning both of you in a beautiful bubble of white or golden light, and flutter your eyes open when you are ready. No matter where you are, you can reconnect to this feeling by simply slowing your breath and remembering the image that you have of the feeling of love for your baby.

Mommy Move

Reverse Warrior on a Chair

The warrior stories in the practice of yoga are all about standing your ground and feeling your power. This particular variation is sometimes called Reverse Warrior, and others, including me, refer to it as Exalted Warrior. The second name reflects the energy of the pose. You can envision yourself as the victorious warrior mama who is lifting her heart and her gaze to the sky and feeling the awe-inducing power of the female body. You are literally able to hold space for a whole new person to come into this world. This posture is a variation of Warrior 2, in which you are supported by a chair. Here's how to do this pose.

1. Begin by sliding your left leg through the back space of a chair, so that you can straddle the chair sideways.
2. Bend your left knee to 90 degrees and straighten your back leg with the outer edge of your foot pressing down into the floor.
3. Sweep your left arm up to the sky and let your right hand rest gently on your right leg (see figure).
4. Easily turn your gaze toward the sky unless you have neck pain, in which case your gaze can be down and back over the right shoulder.
5. Breathe deeply and work toward sustaining the pose for about 60 to 90 seconds. Repeat on the other side.

Information No One Tells You

Finding a Comfortable Sleep Position

Insomnia during pregnancy is very common. The dramatic shifts in hormonal levels can cause insomnia, as can finding a comfortable sleep position. For moms who were belly sleepers before pregnancy, it can be especially challenging to find a comfy resting position. It is generally recommended that pregnant women sleep on their left side or on their back with pillows that create an incline (head above the heart, heart above the hips). Lying on the left side allows for proper venous return for mama and in turn for baby. Depending on which you prefer, there are two different types of pillows that can be very helpful during pregnancy. The first type of pillow has several names: Snoogle, boyfriend pillow, body pillow. This pillow is long and narrow and is great for mamas who prefer to sleep on their side. It is better for the used-to-be belly sleepers too, as you can place it between your knees and wrap it under the left side of your tummy so that you have the side of your tummy on the pillow. Granted, it is not the same as lying on your tummy, but for safety reasons, this is as close to that as possible. The second type of pillow is a backrest pillow.

Sometimes called a wedge, this pillow was popular many years ago for watching TV. It is easy to find on Amazon, or from any retailer that offers lots of different pillow options. Many of them come with a plush cover that has side pockets where you can tuck a remote control or snacks. This pillow keeps your head upright, so if that is new or strange to you, maybe save it for watching TV or working on your laptop.

Both these types of pillows are useful after pregnancy too. The body pillow can be wrapped into a horseshoe shape and your baby can use it for tummy time (after six or seven months, when baby can lift head easily), or to lie on the back when head and neck control has been achieved. The backrest pillow can also be used for back support when you are nursing or bottle-feeding baby.

Love-Your-Baby Visualization

Connecting to Your Inner Vision

Merriam-Webster defines *visualization* as the "formation of mental visual images." The act of visualizing is often referred to in sports psychology. For example, a basketball player might prepare for a game by closing the eyes and envisioning the ball going into the basketball hoop many times. The body–mind connection is such that the effect of mentally rehearsing can improve the athlete's performance. The same technique can be used to create your vision of what you would like to have happen during labor and delivery. Just as in the athlete's case, preparing for the intense physical event of having a baby can be beneficial. Whether you are having a scheduled C-section or are preparing for a vaginal delivery, it's good to allow your body and mind to have the mental rehearsal of feeling strong, empowered, and loved.

Begin this visualization by seeing yourself in the labor and delivery room, whether that is in a hospital, a birthing center, or your living room. Take a moment to identify who is going to be in the room, such as a family member or friend, an ob/gyn, a midwife, or a doula. In your mind's eye, envision each of these individuals gazing at you with encouragement and positive energy. Now turn the attention to your own face in this imaging, and feel a gentle smile across your lips, knowing that you are completely supported by the team around you. Feel the confidence and security in your body and how that brings about a sense of empowerment. You can take this visualization all the way forward in time, to the first time that you hold your baby in your arms. Connect to the amazing feeling of joy that fills you as you gaze into your little one's eyes for the very first time. When you feel a sense of completion, gently flutter your eyes open. This visualization can be practiced at any time, as many times as you wish.

Fun Foods

In many esoteric traditions, it is believed that by consuming food that is the same color as a chakra you help nourish that energy center too. That might sound a little out there, but we know from extensive research on nutrition that eating natural foods in a variety of colors helps to give us a wide array of benefits. In fact, many toddler plates come with colors and pictures of green vegetables, red or orange

> continued

fruits, and brown or tan whole grains. Here is an easy way to prepare vegetables, inspired by the rainbow.

Grilled Rainbow Veggies

   Oil for coating veggies

   1 cup asparagus, whole and trimmed

   4 small carrots, cut in half lengthwise

   1 small red pepper, cut into 1-inch strips

   1 medium yellow summer squash, cut into 1/2-inch rounds

   1 medium red onion, cut into wedges

   Salt and pepper

Drizzle vegetables with oil and transfer them to a grill basket. Grill over medium heat for 12 minutes. Season to taste with salt and pepper.
Yield: *4 servings*

Prepare for Birth and Beyond

4

First Trimester: Increase Endurance

During pregnancy, every day is an adventure. Changes in your body, your mind, and your emotions can occur daily. Information is powerful, and it's helpful to learn about the enormous changes that are happening in your body during the first trimester. No two pregnancies are alike, even for the same mom, but there are some common themes during each trimester. Fatigue is often present during this period because of all of the physical changes in your body. Integrating some simple techniques for endurance can help to ease the fatigue. I know it sounds counterintuitive to work out when you are fatigued, but a little bit of gentle exercise can help increase your energy.

Your Body in the First Trimester

During the first trimester, there are some days when we feel absolutely fantastic, even goddesslike, as we realize that the potential to bring life into this world is beginning. On other days, we just want to take a nap—like, all day! Try to be gentle with yourself and remember that this is all par for the course. There is so much happening in the body of a mother that it is completely natural and normal to feel fatigued.

Because you will have more energy some days than others, it is important to be patient with your body and practice compassion for yourself. I often remind pregnant mamas-to-be that they are working harder than anyone else in the room even while simply sitting down. During the first trimester, the baby's neural tube is developing, and by the end of the third month, it already has little hands, little feet, and a functioning liver. So please remember to be kind to yourself and stay receptive to the feedback of your body. The messages from the body during pregnancy are not subtle; sometimes it is screaming for rest. If you need to rest, please honor that. If you feel like you have a little bit of energy and would like to work with that energy in a softer way, choose the Steady As She Goes practice in this chapter, which is gentle in nature. This program integrates a very short standing sequence and is fantastic for those days when you would prefer most of the practice to be seated or lying down.

On other days you will have more energy, and this is the time to increase your endurance. Endurance is a necessary tool throughout pregnancy, labor, and delivery, and beyond. In my experience with thousands of women, the physical endurance that we cultivate in class often converts to mental and emotional endurance as well. We know from the world of sports psychology that the brain often gives up before the body needs to. In this case, try working with positive thoughts like *I am building endurance right here, right now*. Mental imagery can be beneficial as well. Envision your body getting stronger with each breath, each movement, and imagine that you are sharing that strength with the little one inside you. On the days when the energy and motivation are there, try the Let Your Light Shine program (more about this later in this chapter.

Fatigue is not the only feeling you might experience during your first trimester. There might be a lot of what parents of toddlers call *big feelings*—having an emotion overtake you, such as crying at a diaper commercial. This too is totally normal and is a result of the hormonal fluctuations in your body. The increase in estrogen can make your moods shift, while the increase in progesterone can make you constipated and bloated. Progesterone in particular slows down the function of smooth muscle (aka digestion), and that can lead to some tummy trouble. With all of these changes happening, you might be wondering *How am I supposed to work out?*

Many women ask if it is safe to work out during the first trimester, or if they can continue to do what they were doing before pregnancy. Mamas-to-be might ask about everything from *Is it safe to do handstands?* to *What about running sprints?* There are as many opinions about exercise as there are sources, so how is a mindful mama to know what is true? First off, with any exercise program, it is important to have clearance for exercise from your obstetrician or midwife. Ob/gyns and other trained birth professionals will assess whether you have a high-risk pregnancy and what the implications for exercise might be. If you are not categorized as high risk, and are given the green light to exercise, there are many forms of exercise you can continue to enjoy.

The most basic rule for the first trimester is (yes, I'm going to keep emphasizing this): If you were not participating in the activity before you were pregnant, now is not the time to start. This rule, like so many rules during pregnancy, has an exception, and that exception is prenatal yoga. Obviously if you have chosen to begin a yoga practice for the first time during pregnancy, you will not be attending a level 2 or level 3 vinyasa flow class and learning headstands. But there is so much in the prenatal yoga practice that can leave you feeling refreshed and revitalized, especially during the first trimester, that you may find it particularly helpful.

Motivation for Moms

A good place to start any prenatal fitness program is with motivation and inspiration. When we know the Why for exercise, we are much more likely to stick with a program, especially on the days when our energy is a little bit low. Here are some of the many benefits of exercise during pregnancy for you and your baby.

How Prenatal Maternal Exercise Benefits You

- Increases energy, feelings of well-being.
- Promotes a positive self-image.
- Strengthens your heart and blood vessels.
- Strengthens muscles in preparation for labor and support.
- Reduces back pain.
- Eases constipation.
- Improves posture and biomechanics.
- Improves circulation.
- Increases flexibility.
- Improves your overall general fitness.
- Increases or maintains aerobic capacity (endurance).
- Decreases muscle tension, which promotes relaxation.
- Reduces recovery time.
- Promotes healthy weight gain during pregnancy.
- Helps you lose the baby-weight after your baby is born.

How Prenatal Maternal Exercise Benefits Your Baby

- Regular maternal exercise throughout gestation results in significantly lower fetal heart rate (HR) and increased heart rate variability (HRV).
- Exercise supports appropriate fetal body weight and composition, cardiovascular health, and nervous system development.
- Exercise during pregnancy may elicit a prenatal programming effect, creating a healthy environment in utero during a critical time of organ development.
- There is evidence that women who exercise while pregnant have calmer babies who sleep better.

In addition to these benefits, maternal exercise can also help decrease the risk of the following.

- Edema (swelling)
- Fatigue
- Insomnia
- Gestational diabetes
- Diastasis recti (abdominal separation)
- Pelvic and rectal pressure
- The need for surgical or medical interventions
- Postpartum weight retention
- Depression

Exercise during pregnancy has so many benefits that you might want to photocopy these lists and tape them to your bathroom or kitchen cabinet. Starting each day with a powerful list of benefits can help you to remember some of the Whys for your exercise program. Use a highlighter on the points that are especially important to you, and write in additional words of motivation like *You've got this, mama!* Staying motivated to exercise will help keep you on track with your daily program.

Exercise in the First Trimester

Now that you know the reasons why it's great to move, let's look at how to begin. Whether you are a workout queen or have let go of your fitness routine for a while, meditation is a great place to begin. Meditation will help you set an intention and keep your mind focused. Yoga is the next step, or bridge, to strong movement. Your practice can be as light or as challenging as you need on any given day so it allows you to work around the first trimester challenges like nausea and fatigue. Yoga uses the weight of your body as resistance and is a natural segue into strong fitness moves like squats and lunges. Keeping up your strength, flexibility, and cardiovascular endurance are all beneficial during pregnancy. The Mothers Into Living Fit 3 + 1 model provides a well-rounded, holistic approach to movement throughout your pregnancy. Here's a deeper look into each component.

Meditation

An integral part of the practice, and a wonderful place to begin your health and fitness program, is with meditation. Meditation does not have to be scary or intimidating. It is not necessary to chant *om* for an hour while seated in Lotus Pose. Meditation simply refers to silencing all of the mental chatter in our minds and connecting to a deep sense of center. This practice can be tremendously beneficial to both mother and baby during pregnancy.

In his book *Magical Beginnings* Deepak Chopra tells us that the unborn baby can feel everything the mother feels and that the baby has its own unique nervous system. This means that if the mama is stressed (traffic, bad day at work, etc.), then the baby has its own fight-or-flight reaction to the situation. The baby has nowhere to go, so it is flooded with stress hormones like cortisol, which can lead to lower birth weight. Conversely, babies of mothers who practice meditation are bathed in feel-good chemicals like endorphins and encephalins. Meditation during the first trimester can be a wonderful way to connect to your inner voice and start your day with a sense of peace, calm, and centeredness.

Many yogis meditate at dawn. Meditating first thing in the morning is a sweet way to transition from the dream state into the rest of the day. When you meditate before you have checked email and social media or watched the morning news, there has been no input from the outside world. It is during this quiet time in the morning that you can hear yourself think, and start the day the way you choose to rather than in reaction to outside news. Here is a quick morning meditation to start your day feeling centered and energized.

Before you even open your eyes in the morning, take a moment to slow your breath down and feel your energy levels. Envision a beautiful golden light in your belly, the color of sunshine. With each inhalation, envision that light growing more radiant, like the rays of the sun. Sense, see, and feel that light radiating out to your arms, legs, fingertips, and toes. Breathe into the feeling of being completely luminous and filled with the warmth of the sun. When you feel a sense of completion, slowly flutter your eyes open and begin your day.

Yoga

In addition to meditation, a gentle yoga practice is an effective way to connect with your body during pregnancy. Yoga can help with your posture, your circulation, and your energy levels. During the first trimester, a strong workout simply might not be possible. There is so much happening inside your body, and chances are there is fatigue as a result of the internal changes. Your body is working hard even when you are at rest. A gentle yoga practice allows you to *meet your body where it is now*. This simply means that if your body is tired, it is not time for burpees and sprints. Exercises that move slowly and mindfully and provide a foundation of strength are better suited to the first trimester. Yoga can help with your energy levels because

Special Instructions for Prenatal Yoga

Please be aware that just as there some poses in the practice of yoga that are absolutely amazing during pregnancy, there are some that need to be avoided (aka contraindicated) throughout the entire pregnancy, including the first trimester. As soon as pregnancy is confirmed, you should avoid Cobra, Bow, Locust, Forward Fold with legs together, all deep twists, and breath of fire.

In addition, there are special instructions for yoga during pregnancy. Please remember that in addition to this list, if there is anything that just feels wrong, immediately let go of that pose.

- Get your doctor's clearance before starting any exercise program.
- Have regular checkups to ensure the health of the baby and of the placenta.
- Keep your head above your heart most of the time (Forward Folds can be modified).
- Avoid deep Forward Folds, and widen your stance for modified Forward Folds.
- Avoid deep twisting and twists where you cross the midline of the body.
- Avoid prone (on the belly) exercises.
- Avoid supine (flat on the back) exercises after the first trimester; brief (less than 90 seconds) work may be okay.
- Be careful not to overstretch or move too deep into a posture.
- Breathe deeply (if ujayii, or diaphragmatic, breathing is not comfortable, breathe naturally).
- Stop immediately if you experience any dizziness or bleeding.
- Avoid breath retention and sharp exhalations (kapalabhati, or breath of fire).
- Avoid hot yoga and extreme temperatures, as extremely high maternal core temperature has been linked to problems with the baby's neural tube.

the sequences build slowly from the ground up and can help you maintain your stamina for the duration of your pregnancy. Please don't worry if you are new to yoga or are not sure where to start. Safe yoga postures for the first trimester are included later in this chapter.

Cross-Training

Once you have started working with meditation and yoga to help increase your endurance, you might want to start cross-training. Cross-training means engaging in two or more types of exercise in your exercise program. A great form of exercise that pairs well with yoga for moms-to-be is walking. Walking is part of our daily life, and it is free. Walking can also feel like a moving meditation, and help you clear your mind when there are so many voices giving you advice. Well-meaning friends and relatives often overshare and give a lot of details about their own labor and delivery. Walking is a wonderful opportunity not only to get fit but also to check in with your own inner wisdom and let go of outside opinions. Plus, walking is a sweet opportunity to have an inner dialogue with your baby, or perhaps to start to daydream about what your life will be like when your baby is in your arms. Allow yourself to feel the joy of movement with your baby, and move toward a state of flow.

Flow—a term often used in sports psychology—was coined in the 1990s by a psychology professor named Mihaly Csikszentmihalyi. He described the flow state as "being completely involved in an activity for its own sake. The ego falls away. Time flies. Every action, movement, and thought follows inevitably from the previous one, like playing jazz. Your whole being is involved, and you're using your skills to the utmost." For pregnant mamas, walking as a method to tap into flow can be very rewarding. It is often during these times that we have what Oprah calls an *aha moment*. These moments of realization can be as simple as *My body feels great when I move, and I know that this is helping prepare me for motherhood* to a realization that *I want to be very protective of my energy right now. I am making a baby, and healthy boundaries are good. I don't have to say yes to everything and everyone.*

This is how we allow our physical strength to help build our mental and emotional strength. Simply shifting the focus can help prepare our bodies, minds, and hearts for motherhood. I can hear some of you thinking, *A strong mind and state of flow sound great, but what about my booty? Will all of this walking help lift my rear view?* The answer is a resounding Yes! According to researchers at the Mayo Clinic, a regular walking program can help you

▮ maintain a healthy weight,

▮ prevent or manage various conditions, including heart disease, high blood pressure and type 2 diabetes,

▮ strengthen your bones and muscles,

▮ improve your mood, and

▮ improve your balance and coordination.

Quick Note on Cardio and Eating

Now is not the time to try to manage your caloric intake with what I call *punishment exercise*. This refers to overeating at a meal and then promising yourself to compensate for that meal with a tremendous amount of exercise, usually cardio. We have all done it at one time or another, perhaps after Thanksgiving dinner or Super Bowl snacks. Eating during pregnancy, like exercising, should be balanced. Your caloric needs will modestly increase in the first trimester. It is not unusual for pregnant mamas to find that they crave foods from their childhood. PB and J, mac and cheese, even Pop-Tarts might be calling your name. If there is an overwhelming craving for carbohydrates, it makes sense. During the first trimester, you are making little fingers, toes, and a skeletal system within your womb. That requires extra energy in the form of calories, and very often from carbohydrates. Try eating more complex carbohydrates like steel-cut oatmeal with a little bit of organic peanut butter to add some fat and protein. This will prevent your blood sugar from rapidly spiking and then crashing. Celebration eating and punishment exercise can leave you feeling depleted; this is not a sustainable or balanced way of nourishing your body, especially during pregnancy. Taking the extra time to plan your meals a day or two in advance will help you to avoid overeating and being tempted to overexercise.

Some of the muscles that a walking program can strengthen are the hamstrings and the glutes. These muscles will be more toned, which not only looks good but can lead to better posture during pregnancy. Later in the pregnancy, when baby is growing and pulling the abdomen forward, the lower back compensates by contracting and often feels tight. At the same time, the hip flexors can get tight while the hamstrings can become lax. We will explore posture in greater detail later in this chapter. For now, please know that walking can help strengthen the muscles that will give you better posture throughout your pregnancy.

Walking is a very effective form of cardiovascular exercise and is a great complement to your yoga practice. Cardiovascular exercise is any exercise that increases your heart rate. You might already be feeling the increase in the demands on your heart and lungs. During pregnancy, your body carries up to 50 percent more blood volume. If you find yourself starting to breathe a little bit heavier when walking up a few stairs, that is completely normal. Walking is a great form of cardio to enjoy while pregnant because you can easily gauge what level of effort you should give, based on your body's response. Here are some tips to make the most of your walking program.

- Invest in good shoes; your feet might grow during pregnancy, and they need proper support.
- Invest in a good sports bra; there should be ample support and two separate built-in cups.
- Bring a water bottle; in addition to your own hydration needs, the placenta needs H_2O.

▌ Stand tall during your walking program, similar to Mountain Pose in yoga.

▌ Walk at a slower pace for at least two minutes before increasing your pace.

▌ Phone apps and activity trackers are a great way to track your steps for the week.

▌ Remember that there are benefits from as little as 10 minutes of walking.

▌ Break up the workout if necessary, for example, a 10-minute morning walk and a 10-minute afternoon or evening walk.

▌ Walk at a pace that allows you to be able to carry on a conversation, but not so easy that you can sing.

▌ In the case of extreme cold or extreme heat, walk indoors on a treadmill or at the mall.

▌ Bring your cell phone in case of emergency, and let someone know where you will be walking.

▌ Listen to your body and rest if necessary.

▌ Have fun and talk to your baby; you have a built-in training partner who loves your voice.

The CDC (Centers for Disease Control) recommends that pregnant women walk 150 minutes a week. That sounds like a lot, but remember that it's totally fine to break up your workouts into two separate windows of exercise, as indicated in the list you've just read. Walking for 10 minutes in the morning can help you wake up, connect to your breath, connect to your baby, and set you up for success, meaning that you are more likely to meet your exercise goals if those goals are tangible and realistic. Setting smaller, manageable goals is a good choice throughout pregnancy.

Yoga Poses and Exercises for the First Trimester

The following poses will help you maintain endurance during the first trimester. There are cues for enjoying each pose throughout your pregnancy. Move slowly, breathe deeply, and enjoy your yoga practice.

Easy Pose

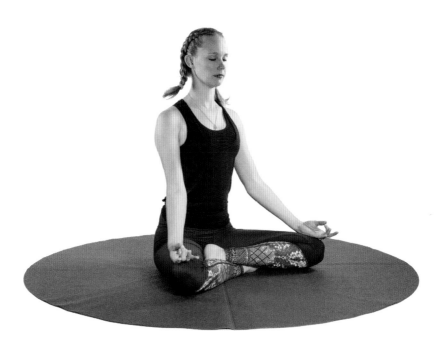

Benefits

This pose is a very gentle opener for the hips and also invites a sense of ease.

Feeling

The pose brings a feeling of peace and tranquility.

Instruction

- Begin seated and cross your legs in the way that is most comfortable for you with either the right or left leg in front.
- Sit up straight and feel length in your side body (waist).
- Lengthen your neck and allow your shoulders to move easily down and away from your ears by relaxing the trapezius muscles (see figure).

Adjustments

Easy Pose can be practiced with your back against a wall if you are feeling very fatigued. If you are in Easy Pose for an extended period (especially for meditation), sitting on top of a blanket or two can feel very comfortable.

Unicorn and Rainbow Pose

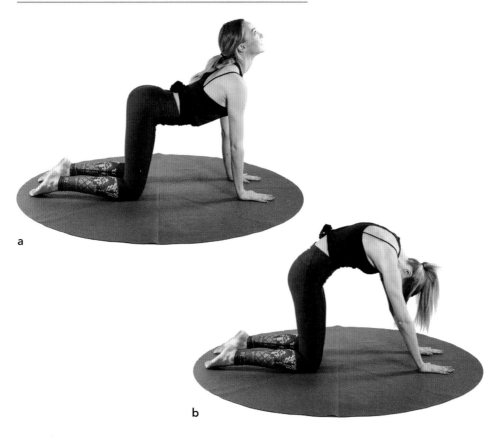

a

b

Benefits

This pose sequence, often called cat and cow, helps to strengthen and maintain flexibility in the lower back and abdomen.

Feeling

This sequence is a very gentle way to warm the core muscles. Invite the feeling of warmth from the inside out.

Instruction

▮ Begin on all fours with hands shoulder width apart and knees hip width apart.
▮ Inhale and gaze to the sky, lifting the breastbone and the coccyx (tailbone) toward the sky as you softly contract in your lower back (see figure a).
▮ Exhale and round the spine in the shape of a rainbow. Take it easy with the pelvic tuck in the second and third trimesters, and focus more on the curve in the upper body (see figure b).

Adjustments

You can use a folded blanket under your knees to cushion them. Or you can practice this sequence standing, with feet hips width apart, a soft bend in the knees, and hands on top of the thighs.

Pointer Dog Pose

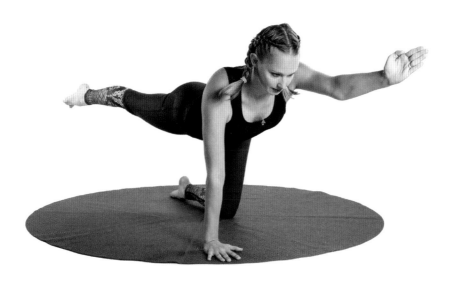

Benefits

This pose is great for core strength (TVA, obliques, lower back) and is also beneficial for balance training.

Feeling

This gives you a long line of energy extending in two directions (front and back), like the arrow on a compass.

Instruction

▌ Begin on all fours with hands shoulder width apart and knees hips width apart.
▌ Inhale and lift your left arm with the thumb pointed to the sky and your right leg to the height of the hip.
▌ Find length in the spine as you reach the front hand away from the back foot and feel a gentle lift in the abdomen, so that there is muscular support under the pose (see figure).
▌ Keep your neck long with the gaze about 12 inches ahead of the yoga mat.
▌ Enjoy three to five deep breaths, and then change sides.

Adjustments

You can use a folded blanket under your knees to cushion them. If there is *any* pulling in the abdomen, lower your back toes to the ground. If there has been a lot of round ligament pain during this particular time of gestation, it is recommended that you keep the back foot on the floor the entire time.

Down Dog Pose

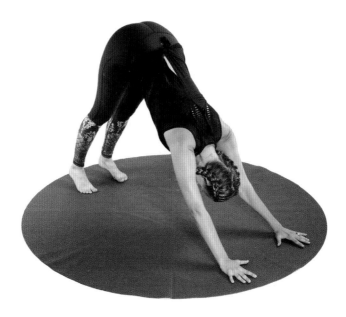

Benefits

This pose (aka Downward-Facing Dog) is a wonderful stretch for the entire back of the body from head to toe. Down Dog is also considered an inversion because the head is below the heart, and the heart is below the hips. Inversions help to bring oxygenated blood to the brain as well as giving a new perspective on the world.

Feeling

Down Dog is a gentle inversion, and often feels fantastic during pregnancy. Allow yourself to connect with the energy of Mother Earth and feel her rising up to support you and your baby.

Instruction

- Begin on all fours with hands shoulder width apart and knees hip width apart.
- On your exhalation, lift your hips to the sky with straight arms and straight legs. Be aware that the elbows and knees are soft, not locked (see figure).
- If you are in your second or third trimester, it can often feel much more comfortable to have the stance wider. It is fine to have the feet as wide as the yoga mat; just make sure that when you look back at your feet you are looking at your toes, and that the heels are barely visible, because they are tilting slightly outward as a result of internal rotation in the hip joint.

Adjustments

Remember that, depending on how you are feeling that day, Down Dog may or may not feel great. If you have nausea, heartburn, or wrist pain, consider skipping this pose for the time being and enjoying stability on all fours instead, especially in vinyasa, or flow, sequences.

Mountain Pose

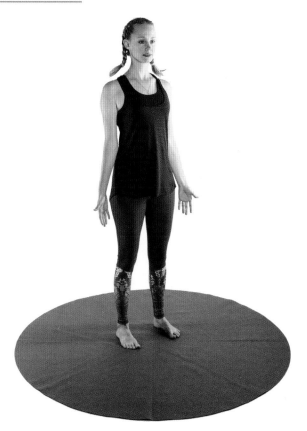

Benefits

This pose teaches correct posture, especially during pregnancy.

Feeling

There is a wide base of support with the head lifted toward the sky, inviting the energy of the mountains. It can be helpful to close your eyes for a breath or two and envision a beautiful mountain and consider how your body is creating the shapes found in and inspired by nature.

Instruction

- Stand with feet hip width apart and a slight bend in the knees.
- Feel your spine lengthen and the crown of your head rising up toward the sky.
- Gently firm your thighs and lengthen your tailbone down toward the floor.
- Allow your arms to lengthen at your sides and turn the palms to face forward as a result of a soft external rotation at the shoulder (see figure).

Adjustments

During the latter part of the pregnancy, it is especially important to be aware of posture and engage a very light contraction in the abdomen as you exhale. This pose can also be practiced with the arms reaching high to the sky.

Half Forward Fold

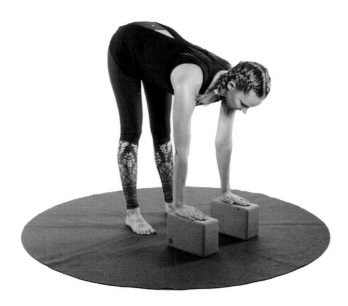

Benefits

This pose is a safe way to train the strength of the lower back as well as the functional skill of lengthening the spine any time you bend over to pick something up.

Feeling

In yoga, the lower back is considered to be very important; in fact, it is said to be the root of the tree of life. The sacrum (the wide bone of the spine toward the bottom), meets the pelvis and creates what is called the sacroiliac, or SI, joint. The word *sacrum* has the same root as the word *sacred*; many yogis consider this area to be the beginning of life. Consider envisioning your lower back as a source of strength and sense, see, and feel the muscles as a powerful tool for carrying the weight of the pregnancy in a comfortable way.

Instruction

▌ Standing with feet hip width apart, put a gentle bend in the knees so that they are not locked.

▌ Hinge forward and place your fingertips on blocks at the desired height (they should be tall enough so your head and your tailbone can be in alignment).

▌ Let the back of the head and neck stay long, with your gaze about 12 inches in front of the blocks (see figure).

▌ Be aware that your body weight is pitched forward slightly so you are not sitting back into the heels.

Adjustments

Gently drawing the shoulders back and away from the ears can help to lengthen the neck. Also, remember that blocks are intended to fill in the space between you and the floor. During the latter part of the pregnancy, it will often feel much more comfortable to have the blocks on their tallest side.

Sun Salutations to Start Your Day

On days when you do not have time for a full practice, an easy and quick morning practice can gently help you wake up and set the tone for the day. With sun salutations, you welcome the energy of the new day and all of the infinite possibilities it can bring. Sun salutes help you gently warm up the body, including the muscles that support respiration, so you can enjoy a deeper breath. As your pregnancy progresses, it can sometimes feel like you are a little bit short of breath, especially if you have a short torso and there is not as much space for a full diaphragmatic breath. Enjoying a quick series of three Sun Salutations can be a great way to start the day.

Sun Salutations also help us invite the solar qualities of light and radiance. The ancient yogis designed several variations, which help to warm up the larger muscle groups through forward flexion (bending forward), back extension (bending backward), as well as movements that are familiar in fitness classes, like squat position, lunge, and triceps push-up (Chaturanga). During pregnancy, many of these poses need to be modified to keep a safe space for your baby. There are some varying opinions on the actual Sun Salutation modifications for pregnancy. I tend to err on the side of caution and make sure that you have options for the days that you feel very strong as well as for the days when you might need an easier option.

Since there are many different forms of Sun Salutation, they are often given letter designations. For our purposes, I have integrated three versions into your program design to invite strength and a feeling of bright energy: Half Sun Salutation, Sun Salutation A, and Sun Salutation B. You will find detailed instructions for the Half Sun Salutation and Sun Salutation A in the next section of this chapter; Sun Salutation B is described in detail in chapter 5.

Half Sun Salutation

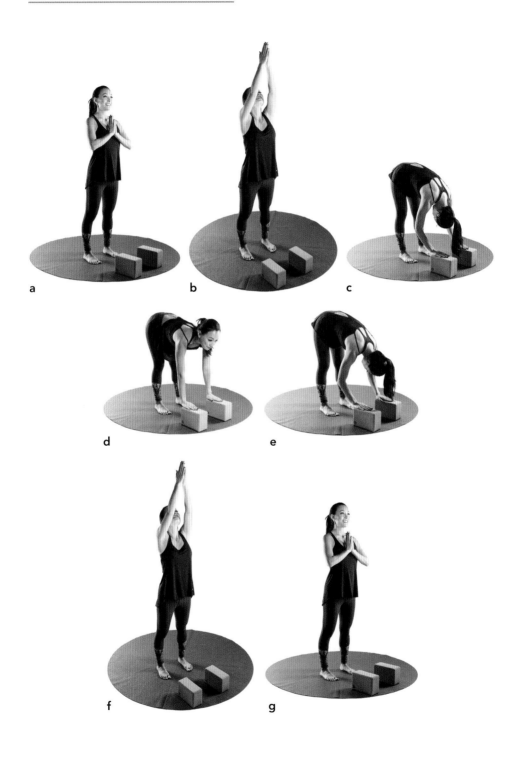

Benefits

This sequence warms up the upper body in a very gentle way as well as bringing the feeling of stability to the legs and the lower body.

Feeling

Consider inviting the warmth of the sunrise and the possibilities of the new day with each round of Sun Salutation. Breathe in the feeling of warm, pleasant sunshine, and share that with the baby inside you.

Instruction

- Begin in Mountain Pose with the feet hip width apart and all ten toes pointing directly forward (see figure a).
- On the inhalation, come into Mountain Pose with the arms up by raising the arms to the sky, and feel length in the spine (see figure b).
- On the exhalation, come into a modified or soft version of Forward Fold by gently folding forward with hands on blocks and a soft bend in the knees (see figure c).
- Inhale and rise up halfway with a long flat spine, and hands supported by the blocks into Half Forward Fold (see figure d).
- On the exhale, softly bow the head and neck (see figure e).
- Inhale and rise all the way up to standing with the arms reaching out like wings and hands meeting at the top (see figure f).
- Finish the sequence where you began, in Mountain Pose (see figure g).

Adjustments

Remember that Half Sun Salutation does involve some Forward Folds. Forward Folds during pregnancy look very different than they do in a nonpregnant practice. Keep the knees softly bent and leave space between your feet in all standing work, and especially in Forward Folds. Rather than trying to get as deep as possible (nose to knees), focus more on getting the spine as long as possible. Please consider using the blocks on the tallest optional setting, so as to bring the floor closer to you and take any pressure off the lower back.

Plank Pose

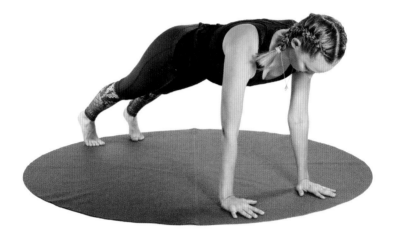

Benefits

This pose maintains strength in the triceps, shoulders, and core.

Feeling

There is a feeling of great strength in the upper body, almost as though you could push the floor away from you.

Instruction

- Begin on all fours with hands shoulder width apart.
- Step one foot back and then place the other into push-up position (see figure).
- Breathe slowly and mindfully, and try to keep your body in a diagonal line. It is important to stay aware that the hips should be neither too high nor too low, as this changes the nature of the exercise. It can be helpful to practice in front of a mirror.

Adjustments

Modified Plank on the knees is a fantastic option if you have wrist pain or feel any pulling in the abdomen, or if you are carrying multiples. Try to keep the amount of time spent in full Plank Pose to a minimum; it's not necessary to be here for long periods of time. The length of three to five deep breaths is ample to reap the benefits. A blanket under the knees can feel great if you have sensitive knees or are practicing on a hardwood floor.

Modified Chaturanga Pose

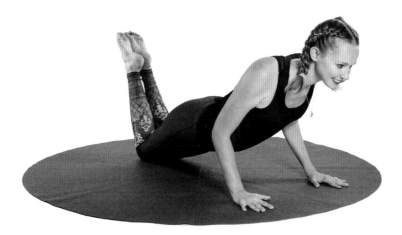

Benefits

This pose, also called Low Plank Pose, strengthens the upper body and the core.

Feeling

You will gain strength, power, and a feeling of hovering above the ground (sort of like a crocodile).

Instruction

- Beginning in modified Plank Pose, feel your elbows point straight back as you bend the elbows only to the point where your belly does not touch the floor, and you feel as though you can safely push right back up to a straight arm (see figure).
- Remember to keep the back of the neck long and the trapezius muscles moving away from your ears.
- It can be very helpful to practice in front of a mirror, or you could take a video of your form to check whether you are in proper alignment.

Adjustments

Padding under the knees can feel great. Please be aware not to lift the hips up too high, as this changes the emphasis of the exercise. Nor should the hips be too low, as that could strain the lower back. Move slowly and mindfully and let your slow, deep breath be an indication that you are practicing at a pace that works for both you and baby.

Sun Salutation A

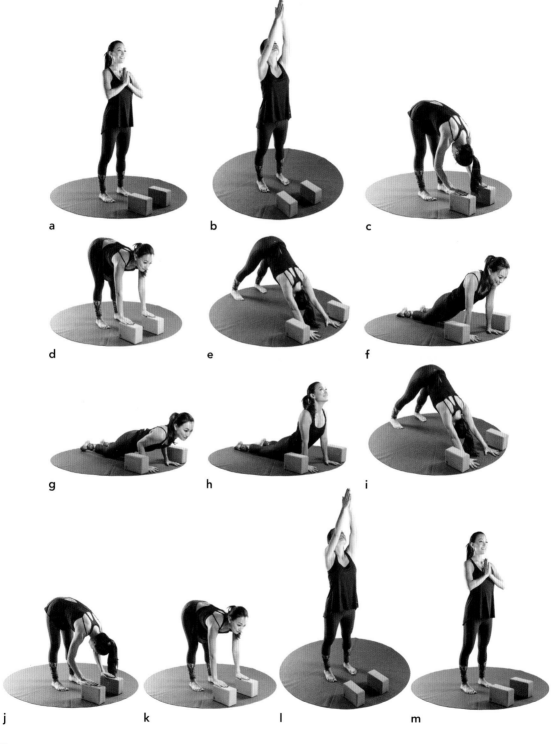

a

b

c

d

e

f

g

h

i

j

k

l

m

Benefits

This sequence helps warm up the entire body and the core.

Feeling

Sun Salutations invite the feeling of sunshine. During full Sun Salutation, take your time in each shape and feel the gentle warmth in the breath and in the body. Let the feeling of warm morning sunshine fill your body with light and radiance.

Instruction

- Begin with feet hip width apart and all ten toes pointing straight forward (see figure a).
- Inhale and raise arms to the sky (Mountain Pose with arms up) as you lengthen the spine (see figure b).
- On the exhalation, enjoy an easy Forward Fold with hands on top of the blocks (remember not to fold in too deep; see figure c).
- Inhale and rise up to a Half Forward Fold with the spine long and the gaze slightly forward, so that the head and neck are an extension of the spine (see figure d).
- Exhale and walk hands onto the floor beside the blocks as you walk the feet back to Down Dog. Enjoy a deep breath in Down Dog as you get your bearings in the inversion (see figure e).
- Inhale and shift forward to a modified Plank with knees on the ground (see figure f). Modify Chaturanga by doing a half push-up, so that the belly never touches the ground (see figure g).
- Inhale into a soft Up Dog or a Unicorn and Rainbow (see figure h).
- Exhale and return to Down Dog, again enjoying a deep breath (see figure i).
- From Down Dog, look forward to your hands and step to the top of the mat into a soft Forward Fold (see figure j).
- Inhale and rise up halfway into Half Forward Fold, feeling length in the spine. Stay in the Half Forward Fold for the exhalation (see figure k).
- On the inhalation, come all the way back up to standing in Mountain Pose (see figure l) with the hands at the heart (see figure m).

Adjustments

There are several ways to adjust this sequence to make it comfortable for pregnancy. Consider having a blanket folded across the middle of the mat so that you have padding for your knees in the modified Plank, or Chaturanga, sequence, as well as for the backbend if you choose Unicorn and Rainbow. When deciding whether to do a soft Up Dog, let your body guide you. There should be no pulling in the abdomen. If there is any feeling of pulling or round ligament pain in Up Dog, choose to drop the knees and enjoy Unicorn and Rainbow instead.

Up Dog Pose

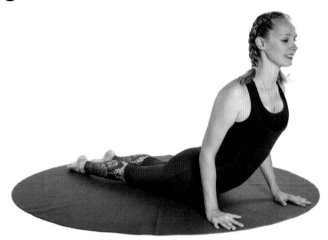

Benefits

This pose (aka Upward-Facing Dog) stretches the chest, the front of the shoulders, and the abdomen. A wonderful tool to help improve posture if there is a tendency to round the shoulders forward, Up Dog can help train the muscles of the midback to draw back and down (scapular retraction and depression).

Feeling

Back bends help us to connect with the feeling of a wide open heart. When we feel scared, nervous, or anxious, the body's natural tendency is to protect the vital organs (the brain and the heart). This can lead to hunching forward as a way to protect the heart space. Feel this space open wide with the new love that is about to enter your life.

Instruction

- From modified Chaturanga, raise your heart to the sky and let your hips softly move toward the floor, but not touching the floor; let them hover above the yoga mat.
- Classically, this pose is practiced with the knees off the floor (see figure). It's OK to let your knees rest on the floor if the stretch in the belly is too deep, or if the pose is a little too challenging with the knees above the floor. The knees-on-the floor variation is sometimes called Swan Pose.
- In either variation, lengthen your neck and press vigorously into your palms to activate the upper arm muscles.
- Breathe deeply and enjoy the feeling of length in the spine and strength in the middle and upper back.

Adjustments

A blanket under the knees or a bolster under the hips, or both, can give additional support. Occasionally this pose does not feel great. If there is diastasis recti from a previous pregnancy, if you are carrying multiples, or if your intuition suggests you should maybe pass on this, consider enjoying the Unicorn and Rainbow Pose instead. Whatever shape you choose, remember that it is not necessary to spend a long time in Up Dog or Swan. A few deep breaths will suffice.

Tree Pose

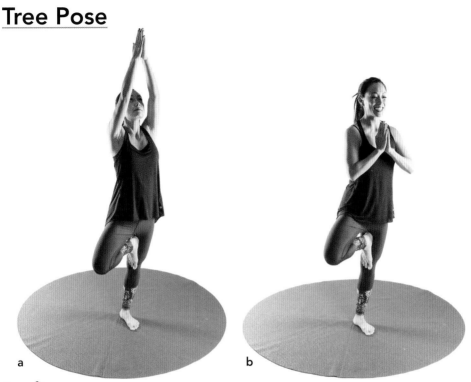

a   b

Benefits

This pose improves balance and increases strength in the standing leg. When practiced with postural awareness, it also benefits the stabilizers of the core.

Feeling

Envision the standing leg as the trunk of a tree and your toes as the roots spreading into the earth. Tap into the feeling of being deeply rooted into the earth's energy as a source of strength, grounding, and support for you and your little one.

Instruction

- Begin standing in Mountain Pose.
- Slowly lift the right foot onto the left inner thigh with the right knee turned out to the right as a result of external rotation of the right hip. (Dancers refer to this external rotation as *turnout*.) Tree Pose has the standing leg in neutral with all five toes pointing straight ahead and the lifted leg turned out (see figure a).
- Bring the hands to the heart center and think about the tailbone pointing down instead of back (see figure b).The idea is to engage your abs lightly so that you are not in a pronounced swayback position.
- Enjoy three to five deep breaths, and then change sides.

Adjustments

Balance is affected by many different factors; lack of sleep, dehydration, emotional state, and pregnancy can all change your sense of balance. Be gentle with yourself, and if it feels better to keep the lifted foot lower, it's OK to place it on the inner calf, or even place the tips of the toes on the floor like a kickstand. If you need additional support with balance, you can place your hand on the wall.

Pigeon Pose

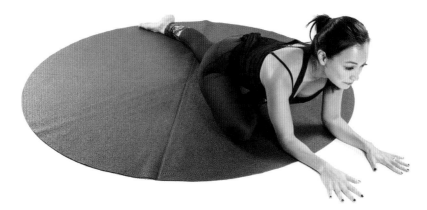

Benefits

This pose is a hip opener that helps to keep hips strong and flexible for labor and delivery.

Feeling

The feeling is one of release, of letting go. It is interesting to note that when a baby exhibits the startle reflex, it is tightening the psoas. This is usually the same area in which adults experience fight-or-flight response. Check in with your breath and simply observe as you come back to the steadiness of the breath.

Instruction

- Begin in a low lunge position with the right foot in front and the left leg extended behind you.
- Slowly, toe-heel move your right foot over to the left side until your right lower leg is at a 90 degree angle.
- Take your time settling into this pose and make sure there is never any weight on your belly at all as you fold forward (see figure). Blocks are a great way to lift the floor up to meet your forearms so you can safely keep your belly above the floor at all times.
- Enjoy several deep breaths, and then change sides. It is very important to stay mindful and to stay connected with your breath. Your slow, deep, relaxed breathing pattern is a great indicator that you are working in a way that is self-aware.
- Please be mindful of your entrance and exit for this pose. Because of the increase in the hormone relaxin during pregnancy, there can sometimes be a little bit of laxity, or looseness, in the pubic joint.

Adjustments

Place a bolster underneath your pelvis so that you have cushion as well as a nice lift for the hip with the bent knees. A blanket under the knee of the straight leg can give some cushion, which feels great if you are working on a hardwood floor. The use of blocks is highly recommended here. Cork blocks are a great naturally sourced product that have some give to them but at the same time are very stable.

IT Band Twist

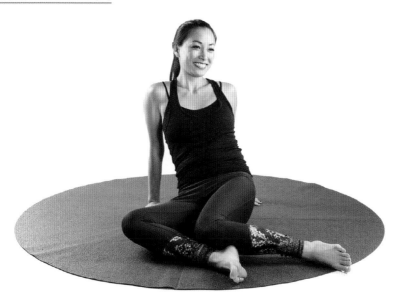

Benefits

This pose stretches the iliotibial (IT) band.

Feeling

Traditional twists are used in the practice of yoga as a kind of palate cleanser. Before moving from hip openers to backbends, for example, it would be common to enjoy a twist. Let this IT band stretch be the replacement for a true twist, and give your body the opportunity to start fresh as you move from one type of stretch into another.

Instruction

- Sit on the floor with feet in front of you and knees bent.
- Cross the right outer ankle in front of the left outer knee, and allow the left inner knee to gently fold down and over to the right (see figure).
- Enjoy three to five deep breaths, come back to the center, and then change sides.

Adjustments

Move slowly and mindfully with this particular stretch. It is contraindicated to move into a deep twist during pregnancy. This is *not* a true twist, but gives the feeling of moving over to the side a bit, and will feel great after hip openers.

Upward-Facing Table Pose

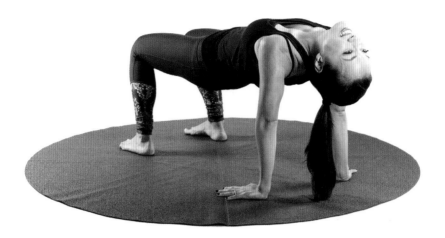

Benefits

This pose opens the top hip and also helps cultivate strength in the back body and the triceps.

Feeling

Root through the hands and invite the feeling of lifting or shining the baby up toward the sky. In the practice of yoga, we often say *root to rise*. This refers to having a strong base of support and pressing into that stable foundation (in this case the hands and feet), in order to enjoy the feeling of rising.

Instruction

- Begin seated in Easy Pose.
- Bring both hands back to about 12 inches behind your hips with the fingertips pointed forward.
- Step one foot forward and then the other with the knees directly over the ankles and all 10 toes pointed straight forward.
- Lift the hips to the sky and find an easy and comfortable place for the head and neck (see figure). Traditionally, the pose is practiced with the head and neck long, as an extension of the spine.

Adjustments

If there is any pain in the head and neck, it's OK to look forward toward your baby. If there is any pain or sensitivity in the wrist or shoulder, it's OK to let the hands turn slightly outward.

Child's Pose

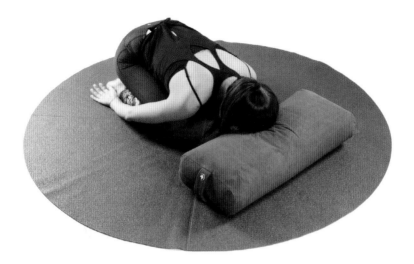

Benefits

This pose helps to promote calm and centeredness.

Feeling

Some teachers call this Wisdom Pose because we must have the wisdom to know when to rest. Knowing when to rest is part of good self-care. As mamas, we model this behavior for our children. Children learn from our actions as much as, or more than, from our words.

Instruction

- Begin on the hands and knees, with knees a little bit wider than the hips.
- On an exhalation, gently bring the hips to meet the heels and reach the hands backward into a comfortable stretch (see figure).
- The forehead will be resting on the earth or on a bolster, and the belly will hover just above the yoga mat (so that it is not bearing weight).

Adjustments

Make sure that the knees are wide enough apart to make space for the baby. If you are carrying multiples, this pose often feels better elevated on bolsters under the forearms; you can also place a blanket across the ankles for comfort.

Upright Hero Pose With Hip Lift

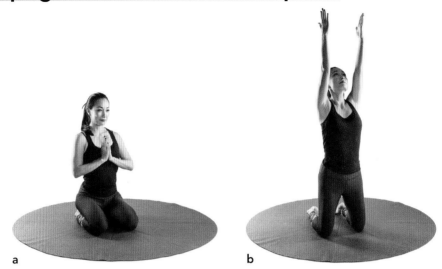

a   b

Benefits

This pose stretches the hips and the groin, elongates the front of the body, and creates a sense of space for a deeper breath as you rise. It provides a gentle warming effect in the entire body, which can help you enjoy a deeper breath because you are also warming the muscles that help to support respiration.

Feeling

You are heroic. Strong. In all poses that have hero energy, remember that you are very much a hero to your baby. Making healthy choices and speaking up for what is right are examples of this energy. For added inspiration, consider the healthy moms and dads who worked hard to create safe car seats. This was a heroic feat; to design something to protect children and have it become the standard is a beautiful example of being a champion for all children.

Instruction

- Begin seated on the knees, with knees hip width apart.
- Be aware that the feet are softly resting straight back on the floor. Try not to roll to the outer arch of the foot, especially if you know that you have a tendency to supinate or if you wear orthotics (see figure a).
- Bring the hands to the heart and on the inhalation rise up tall, circling the arms to the sky (see figure b).
- On the exhalation, draw a line of energy from the sky to the heart and bring the hips back to the heels, in starting position.
- Work up to nine cycles of rising with each inhalation.

Adjustments

During pregnancy, the knees should be a little bit wider than in the traditional pose; this is for safety. Consider practicing with a blanket under the knees for comfort. If the stretch is too intense for the quads, it's OK to practice the sequence seated on a block or two, so that some of the weight is on top of the block. Blocks are also a nice option if your knees are sensitive.

Gate Pose

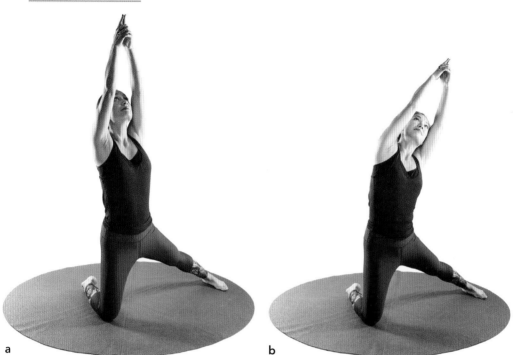

a   b

Benefits

This pose stretches the obliques and the entire side of the trunk. In the practice of yoga, this is often referred to as the *side body*.

Feeling

It can be very sweet to consider the name of the pose and realize that you are stepping through a gateway into motherhood.

Instruction

- Begin kneeling on the floor with the hands at your heart.
- Step the left leg out to the left with the foot pressing gently onto the floor through all four corners of the foot. Reach your arms up to the sky and interlace your fingers with your palms facing inward and your index fingers pointing to the sky (see figure a).
- Bend your upper body to the left as you feel the stretch in the side of your body (see figure b).
- Enjoy three to five deep breaths, and then change sides.

Adjustments

A folded blanket under the supporting knee offers soft cushion. You should also consider the comfort of the head and neck. It's OK to look gently up and continue the energy of the opening toward the sky, but if there is any neck sensitivity you can look down toward the floor. If there is any issue with balance, it's OK to practice with the foot of the outstretched leg propped up on the baseboard of a wall.

Crescent Lunge

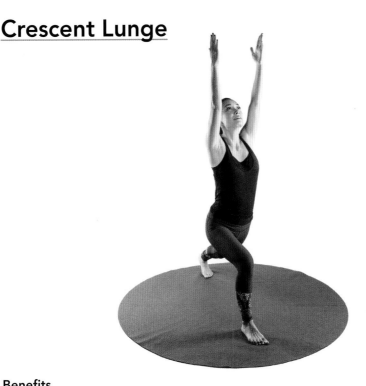

Benefits

This pose opens and stretches the front of the top hip and strengthens the groin, the spine, the pectorals (pecs), and the adductors (inner thighs). It also assists with cultivating balance. This pose may also be called high lunge, low lunge, or low lunge with a lateral hip flexor stretch.

Feeling

The sense is one of rooting to rise; the lower body is strong, grounded, and cultivating stability, while the upper body is rising toward the sky.

Instruction

- From Mountain Pose, step your left foot back into a low lunge position and bend the right knee at a 90 degree angle.
- Feel that the hips are side by side to begin and that the tailbone is gently pointed down toward the earth.
- Sweep both arms up to the sky with your inhalation (see figure), and then interlace the fingers, turning the palms to the sky.
- On the next exhalation, reach up and over to the right, enjoying the stretch in the left psoas and the left side of the waist.
- Enjoy several deep breaths, and then change sides.

Adjustments

The pose can be practiced with the back knee on the floor. A folded blanket under the back knee offers cushion. It's OK to take the stance a little wider from right to left when in the third trimester or if you are carrying multiples. The pose can also be practiced with the arms reaching straight up or leaning in the direction of the front knee for the additional psoas stretch.

Garland Pose

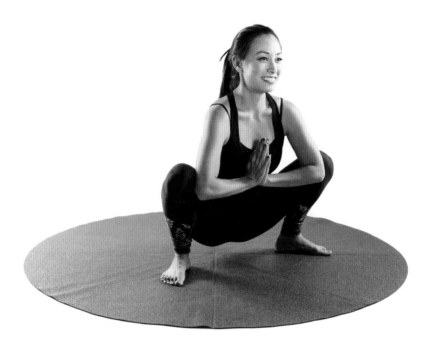

Benefits

This pose assists with the ability to squat, which is often a position chosen for labor and delivery. The natural pull of gravity downward can make delivery in this position easier for many women. The pose also helps improve range of motion of the hip joints.

Feeling

The feeling is one of grounding, of connecting to Mother Earth.

Instruction

- From Mountain Pose, step the feet a little wider than hip width and turn the toes out at a 45 degree angle, hands at the heart.
- Squat down until your hips are hovering above the floor (see figure).

Adjustments

You can place a block or several folded blankets underneath the ischial tuberosities (sit bones) for support. This feels really good, especially if your heels do not easily touch the floor in the deep squat. This position is also great for focusing on pelvic floor strength and can be a great shape for practicing Kegels and other pelvic floor exercises.

Heart-Opening Pose

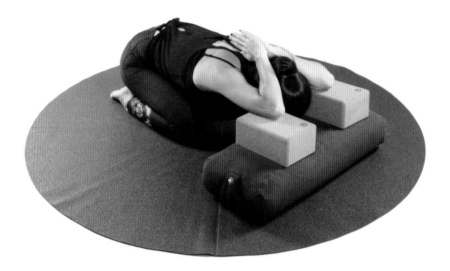

Benefits

This pose provides a deep stretch for the triceps and the shoulders and a very gentle stretch for the front of the torso. It also invites the feeling of opening the heart center.

Feeling

The heart center is the fourth chakra, or energy center, of the body. The primary focus of this center is love. In the pose that is named for the heart center, close your eyes and breathe in the feeling of love to the heart space. Imagine each breath allowing for a sense of expansion, as though you are preparing to meet one of the loves of your life.

Instruction

- Begin on your hands and knees with a bolster in front of you.
- Place two blocks on top of the bolster, with space between the blocks for your head.
- Place your triceps on the blocks and your forehead on the bolster.
- Let the upper body soften into the stretch, completely supported by the blocks and bolster (see figure).

Adjustments

A folded blanket under the knees offers cushion.

Butterfly Pose

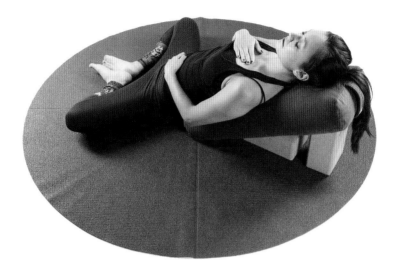

Benefits

This pose provides a passive stretch for the front of the body and the inner thighs. It is effortless and restorative.

Feeling

Feel a sense of surrender, of release, of letting go. This pose is very open and reminiscent of the wings of a butterfly. Allow the butterfly image to be a metaphor for the metamorphosis in your life: becoming a mother.

Instruction

- Begin seated with the soles of your feet together and knees bent.
- Let gravity draw your knees gently down toward the ground and out to the sides like a butterfly's wings.
- I recommend practicing this pose at an incline so that your head is above your heart and your heart is above your hips. This can be done with two blocks, one tall and one short, in a T formation and a bolster placed on top to create an incline pillow. You could also use a few blankets stacked neatly and a bed pillow lying lengthwise on the stack to create an incline pillow. Bring your tailbone to the base of the pillow or bolster and slowly lie down.
- The hands can rest wherever they are most comfortable: at the heart, on your belly, on the earth, or one hand on the heart and one on your baby (see figure).

Adjustments

To make the pose more relaxing, place a folded blanket under the outer knees so that they are completely supported. Or you can roll a blanket and wrap it around your feet. Another sweet option is a lavender eye pillow, and a few drops of citrus essential oil on your wrists.

Deep Relaxation Pose

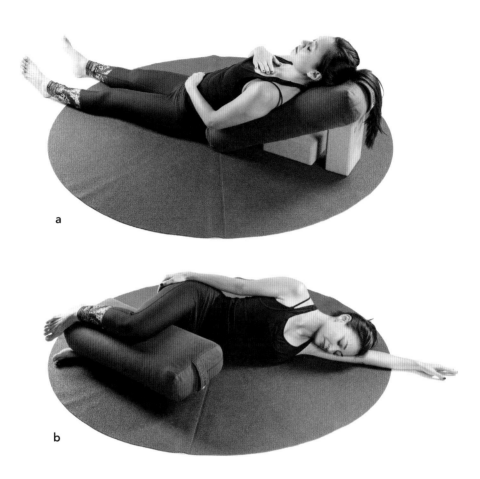

a

b

Benefits

This pose promotes relaxation, softness, and surrender.

Feeling

Allowing Mother Earth to hold the weight of your body, soften completely into this place of comfort and support.

Instruction

- From supported Butterfly Pose, gently stretch your legs to straight.
- Make sure that the feet are at least hip width apart and that the torso is at an incline (see figure a).
- You can straighten the arms down at your sides with the palms facing up.
- Or you can lie on your left side with a bolster or pillow between your knees (lying on the left side allows for proper venous return for mama and in turn for baby), and your head gently resting on your upper arm or on another pillow (see figure b).

Adjustments

This pose is traditionally called Corpse Pose. The idea is to find deep relaxation, letting go of the old while you take time to integrate the new. For pregnancy, I prefer to refer to it as Deep Relaxation. Finding this sense of deep relaxation is personal for each of us. Experiment with what helps you to relax deeply today, such as a lavender eye pillow, aromatherapy, soft music, a blanket covering you, or a partner or spouse massaging your temples.

Putting It All Together

To create a balanced exercise plan for the first trimester, try to include daily meditation and 10 minutes of walking each morning and evening. Then, every other day, choose one of the following two workouts.

There will be days when you feel great and days when you need to take it easy. Let your body's wisdom guide you in your choice of workouts. If you are feeling a bit fatigued, that is completely normal, and it's important to remember that your body is very active even when you are resting. Choose this workout on the days when your body is calling for ease and relaxation. Use this practice during weeks 1 to 12, or until approximately three months.

Exercise	Page	Focus	Reps/Time
Child's Pose	59	Stretches lower back and hips, invites ease	27 slow, deep, centering breaths focusing on the inhalation and the exhalation being equal in length
Upright Hero Pose With Hip Lift	60	Quads and a light warm-up for the cardiovascular system (heart and lungs)	9 rounds of lifting and lowering and marrying that movement to the rhythm of the breath; you can envision a golden circle of light around you and your baby each time you rise
Gate Pose	61	Obliques, adductors, hamstrings	Enjoy 9 deep breaths leaning up and over to the right, take your time during transition, and enjoy 9 deep breaths on the left
Crescent Lunge	62	Psoas and obliques	Enjoy 9 deep breaths leaning up and over to the right, take your time during transition, and enjoy 9 deep breaths on the left
Down Dog Pose	44	Lower back, hamstrings, calves	Work toward 9 deep breaths; if there is nausea, reduce to 3 deep breaths

Exercise	Page	Focus	Reps/Time
Unicorn and Rainbow Pose	42	Lower back and abdomen	9 rounds, inhaling as you gaze up, exhaling as you softly round
Half Sun Salutation	48	Shoulders, core strength and flexibility	3 rounds; remember that each movement corresponds to an inhalation or exhalation
Garland Pose	63	Hips and ankles	9 deep breaths
Heart-Opening Pose	64	Shoulders, pecs, lower back	9 deep breaths
Pigeon Pose	56	Outer thigh, glutes, psoas	9 deep breaths on each side
Upward-Facing Table Pose	58	Lower back, shoulder strength	3 deep breaths
IT Band Twist	57	IT band	3 deep breaths on each side
Butterfly Pose	65	Outer thigh and hip	3 minutes
Deep Relaxation Pose	66	Entire body	3-5 minutes

LET YOUR LIGHT SHINE: FIRST TRIMESTER PRACTICE FOR INCREASING ENDURANCE

There are some days during the first trimester when you feel a little more energetic and might want to build on that feeling of energy. In Sanskrit, *surya* means *sun*; most of the warm-ups are called Sun Salutations. Take your time and stay receptive to the feedback of your body; rest when you need to. Use this practice during weeks 1 to 12, or until approximately three months.

Exercise	Page	Focus	Reps/Time
Easy Pose	41	Gently stretches thighs and invites ease	9 slow, deep, centering breaths focusing on the inhalation and the exhalation being equal in length
Unicorn and Rainbow Pose	42	Warms the abs, TVA, and erector spinae (belly and back)	3 rounds inhaling as you gaze up, exhaling as you round the spine; you can place padding under knees if you wish
Pointer Dog Pose	43	Core stabilization	3 to 5 deep breaths on the right side, pause in the center to find balance, then 3 to 5 deep breaths on the left side
Down Dog Pose	44	Hamstrings, lower back, arm strength	5 slow deep breaths, feeling heels drawn by gravity toward the earth with each breath
Half Sun Salutation	48	Shoulders, core strength and flexibility	3 rounds; remember that each movement corresponds to an inhalation or an exhalation
Sun Salutation A	52	Shoulders, triceps, core strength and flexibility, hamstrings	3 rounds; remember that each movement corresponds to an inhalation or an exhalation

Exercise	Page	Focus	Reps/Time
Tree Pose	55	Inner and outer thigh as stabilizers, core stabilizers	3 to 5 deep breaths on the right, and then left.
Pigeon Pose	56	Outer thighs, glutes, psoas	9 deep breaths on each side
IT Band Twist	57	IT band	3 deep breaths on each side
Upward-Facing Table Pose	58	Outer thighs, glutes, psoas	9 deep breaths on each side
Seated meditation in Easy Pose	41	Gently stretches thighs and invites ease	1 to 3 minutes; sit on a cushion if needed

Mommy Move

Open Door Chest Stretch

The Open Door Chest Stretch is a great stretch for the pecs and the anterior deltoid (shoulder) muscles. These muscles can get tight as a result of what is called *thoracic kyphosis* (aka hunchback). This hunching forward can result from working at the computer or driving, or from the weight and soreness of the breasts as they start to grow, both in size and in sensitivity, from the hormonal shifts of pregnancy. To counteract bad posture, take the time to stretch these muscles at least once a day. This is a very accessible stretch, as it can be done in virtually any open doorway, as outlined here.

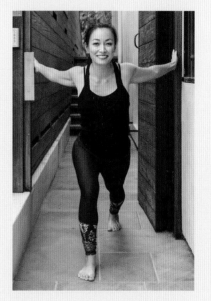

- Place your hands on the sides of the doorframe.
- Step one foot forward and bend the knee slightly so that you can hinge forward comfortably.
- Bring the breastbone forward and keep your spine long (see figure).
- Enjoy 30 to 60 seconds in this stretch while you breathe slowly and deeply.

Information No One Tells You

How Much Caffeine You May Have

As we all know, caffeine is a stimulant. Several studies have examined how much caffeine is safe during pregnancy. Because of conflicting findings, the March of Dimes has stated that pregnant women should limit their daily intake of caffeine to less than 200 mg a day. This is equal to about one 12-ounce cup of coffee. Remember that caffeine can be present not only in coffee but also in tea, sports drinks, and some over-the-counter medications. It's important, therefore, to consider all sources throughout the day, because caffeine does cross the placenta. Babies in utero cannot metabolize caffeine, so it is best to stick with little or no caffeine when possible.

Love-Your-Baby Visualization

Heart-to-Heart Connection

Send your love and blessings from your own heart center to baby's heart center. Close your eyes and slow your breath down. As you breathe, bring your attention to your heart center. The heart center is located at the level of the breasts, in the center of the chest. According to the esoteric teachings, this center corresponds to the color green and to the feeling of love. During pregnancy, many women perceive this heart center energy as a beautiful pink. Whatever color, texture, or feeling you are aware of here, try to connect to what you are holding in your heart for your baby. Compassion, love, excitement, whatever positive feeling you are experiencing, imagine that feeling expanding with each breath. Now envision a beautiful cord of light connecting your heart center to your baby's heart center. Imagine that this cord of light is like an old-fashioned telephone cord, and open the lines of communication. Speak to your baby (silently, internally) and express how much you love him or her (or them, if you are carrying multiples). Let baby feel all of your joy and excitement. Send your love and blessings, the blessings of a mother.

Fun Foods

Ginger is used in the East to help with gastric distress and queasiness. During your pregnancy, ginger tea can help ease nausea throughout the first trimester and beyond. Choose fresh ginger from your local market, and fresh lemon if you need to cut the strong taste of the ginger.

Caffeine-Free Ginger Tea

    1 tablespoon finely grated fresh ginger

    1 cup boiling water

    1 tablespoon freshly squeezed organic lemon juice

    1 tablespoon organic honey

Place the ginger in a medium-sized bowl or teapot. Pour the boiling water over the ginger, letting it steep for at least 5 minutes. While waiting for the tea to steep, put the lemon and the honey into a mug. Strain the ginger when ready, and pour the tea into your mug. Add more lemon and honey as desired.
Yield: *1 serving*

5

Second Trimester: Build Strength

Welcome to the second trimester of pregnancy, which is often called the honeymoon period because most of the fatigue and nausea have typically subsided. You might also notice that your emotions are on a more even keel. Now that you're getting back into the groove of daily life, it's a great time to gently bump up your exercise routine and to focus on building strength. You'll need this strength for the rest of the pregnancy as well as for labor and delivery. Now that you are hopefully feeling your energy levels rising, you have an opportunity to challenge your body a little bit more.

Your Body in the Second Trimester

During the second trimester, your body will start to find a new rhythm and you will probably soon feel your baby's first kicks. Some days you might be feeling like Wonder Woman, ready to tackle any and all challenges. Other days you might feel like your body is a little bit foreign to you, making you wonder *Whose body is this?* Here are some of the changes that might be occurring in your body now.

Weight Gain

Your beautiful baby is getting bigger, and you will start to see your waist getting thicker and your belly pulling forward. Your second trimester body is typically rounder and softer than when you are not pregnant. You will notice that in addition to your abdomen stretching forward, you might have gone up a bra size. Your body is carrying 50 percent more blood volume during pregnancy so there is natural weight gain. In addition to your baby gaining weight and growing, your body is storing fat for breastfeeding. Not to worry; your body is making space for your growing baby, and by maintaining your core strength through safe and intelligent movement, you will be set up for success when you are reclaiming your core strength after labor and delivery. (Note that the beginning of the second trimester is a good time to review all of the safety tips for prenatal exercise in chapter 4!) A pregnant mama's belly is like a house; it is a container of loving, safe space that should never have to bear any external pressure (literally or figuratively). Make sure that you are never lying on your tummy for exercise or sleep. The beautiful sacred space in your belly is growing, and celebrating the changes in your body can help you adapt to your ever-changing body.

Thicker Hair and Glowing Skin

Typically during the second trimester, you will start to notice that your hair is thicker and shinier and there is a natural glow to your skin. There's a shift in your hormone levels; your lush hair is associated with the increase in estrogen, which promotes growth and less shedding. Your glowing skin, also a result of shifting hormones, will often inspire others to compliment you and tell you that you are radiant.

Linea Nigra

Why is there a dark line on my belly? is a common question during the second trimester. As with your beautiful hair and skin, hormonal shifts cause the darkening of the line on your belly, which is called the *linea nigra*, or *black line*. When you are not pregnant, that line on your belly is light and is called the *linea alba*, or *white line*. The linea alba is thick fibrous connective tissue that runs from the base of your breastbone all the way down to your pubis. The darkening of the line on your belly during pregnancy is normal, and usually goes away a few months after your baby is born.

More Energy and Less Fatigue

My energy is coming back is a common statement during the second trimester. Very little in pregnancy is subtle. The changes are often dramatic. But most of the women in my classes, myself included, experience the return of energy levels in a more subtle, gentle way. It can feel as though little by little there is simply more energy. I've heard of women in their first trimester pulling over to the side of the road to catch a quick nap. The second trimester mama still needs plenty of good sleep in the night, but the daytime fatigue often subsides and you can start to get back into your exercise routine.

Exercise in the Second Trimester

Stepping into a second trimester body is a good time to start to find a rhythm to your movement practices, especially if your exercise patterns were a little erratic during the first trimester. It's totally normal for the first trimester to feel like it lacks rhythm with exercise movement, because there are monumental movements and shifts internally. Now that your energy is coming back, it is easier to find a rhythm and establish a regular yoga practice.

With your energy returning, you can also start to build your strength. Physical strength is a tool that can help you carry your pregnancy in a more comfortable way. For example, if your lower back has been achy, building your core strength in a safe and effective way can help with the normal aches and pains of growing a body. The beautiful baby in your belly adds weight to your body, and carrying that extra weight requires strength.

You might have heard the term *functional training* at your gym or from a trainer. Functional training refers to training for a specific task or activity. Pregnancy is unique in that functional training during this special time includes training your body to carry the weight of your baby inside your body. This means that you need to give special attention to the inner unit: the pelvic floor, the TVA, the diaphragm, and the deep muscles along your spine (the multifidi). You are quite literally building your strength from the inside out.

Physical strength can help inspire your mental and emotional strength as well. When you trust your body, it can be easier to feel strong and speak up when you need to. Becoming an advocate for yourself and your baby is an important skill that will serve you well in many situations, including the doctor's office, preschool, and after school activities. The workout called Brave will help you invite the feelings of strength and standing up for yourself and your family when you need to. In the practice of yoga there are many inspirational stories of strength and power, many examples of standing up for what you believe in. One such story is that of Virabhadra (whose name means warrior in English). Virabhadra's is a tragic love story in which he sought to avenge the death of his bride. The story inspired the Warrior yoga poses and demonstrate his actions.

> *Warrior 1* is all about his power and anger rising from the earth.
>
> *Warrior 2* represents the act of drawing his sword, very similar to the stance in fencing.
>
> *Warrior 3* is the act of striking with the sword to seek vengeance for his wife.

In the context of prenatal yoga, we can interpret the symbolism in a slightly different way. Instead of fighting *against* someone or something, we fight *for* what we love. The fierce mama bear energy of protection that rises up in us is undeniable. Many women feel this start to arise during pregnancy. Others feel it more after the baby is born. In either case, mama will move heaven and earth to protect her young. In the second trimester Brave practice, you can invite the feeling of standing your ground into all of the Warrior poses. Beginning to feel the strength of your resolve to protect your little one is a powerful skill you can call on mentally and physically when needed.

Steadiness and Ease

In the practice of yoga, we learn many different concepts that help to inform the physical practice. Yoga has been in existence for centuries, and many of the concepts are timeless. One such concept is called *sthira* and *sukha* which means steadiness and ease. The ancient yogis knew that a steady and easy practice is a sustainable practice. When we try to push too hard or set unrealistic goals, we lose the routine and can feel disheartened as a result. We all know the woman who rarely exercises and then declares on New Year's Day that her resolution is to run 10 miles a day. Such a goal does not set you up for success. A steady, moderate program can leave you feeling energized and motivated to enjoy it again tomorrow.

The key word here is balance. Balancing a few stronger yoga poses with some restorative work at the end can leave you feeling refreshed rather than depleted. You can enjoy this type of practice a few days a week. Just as we find balance in the amount of effort, we can come back to the idea of balancing different forms of movement. It is important to continue to get some regular cardiovascular exercise during pregnancy. Balancing yoga, light weight training, and cardio exercise is a holistic approach to training during pregnancy. I know that sounds like a lot, and you might be thinking, *Hey, wouldn't trying to get in all of those types of exercise make me like the woman who says she's going to run 10 miles a day?* As a trainer, a yoga teacher, and a mom, I have learned some simple techniques to fit it all in.

Fitting It All In

- Lay out your exercise clothes at night for the next day.
- Schedule time for exercise in your phone's calendar and label it *baby time*.
- Exercise for 10 to 20 minutes on days when time is scarce.
- Set up a play mat for toddlers to play yoga with you.
- Invite your friends and family to exercise with you.
- Set an enjoyable place and time for your walks, such as sunset at the beach.
- Create a space in your home for your yoga, such as your living room (store your yoga mat under the couch and have a special candle on the table).
- Keep an extra pair of walking shoes in the trunk of your car.
- Create fun playlists for walking, or listen to audiobooks.

Exercise adherence is the technical term for sticking with your program, and many factors that help to set you up for success are built into these tips. Having a regular appointment with a friend or a trainer is one of the biggest motivators in sticking with your routine. As women, we are very often the caretakers both at work and at home. It is common to put ourselves last on the list, and our own exercise programs can be the first to go when other things need to be taken care of. However, if you have an appointment with someone who is counting on you to be there, you will be much more motivated to show up. An easy way to prioritize your health and yoga practice is to rename it *baby time*. Setting aside time for your own health has benefits for your baby, too. A calm and happy mommy is a huge gift to your little one, both before and after you give birth.

In addition to setting an appointment in your calendar to exercise, planning shorter bouts of exercise can lead to exercise adherence. It is not necessary to exercise for 60 minutes at a time in order to reap health benefits. The CDC recommends at least 150 minutes of exercise a week. This can be broken up into increments of 10- and 20-minute exercise stints, so you can set smaller, attainable goals for movement. Here is a sample schedule for inspiration.

	Sunday	Monday	Tuesday	Wednesday	Thursday	Friday	Saturday
a.m.	20-minute walk	Brave workout	Take It Easy yoga	20-minute walk	Brave workout	Take It Easy yoga	20-minute walk
p.m.	Meditation	20-minute walk	20-minute walk	Meditation	20-minute walk	(Off)	Meditation

Yoga Poses and Exercises for the Second Trimester

The following poses will help you increase your strength during the second trimester. I've included cues for enjoying each pose throughout your pregnancy. Move slowly, breathe deeply, and enjoy your yoga practice.

Sun Salutation B

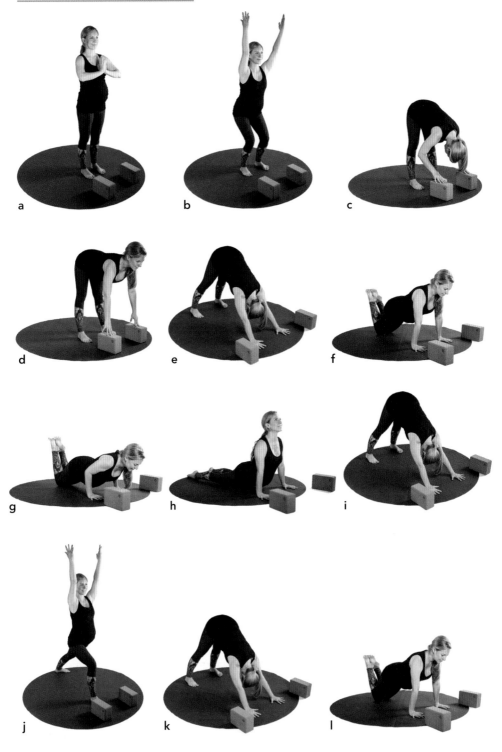

a

b

c

d

e

f

g

h

i

j

k

l

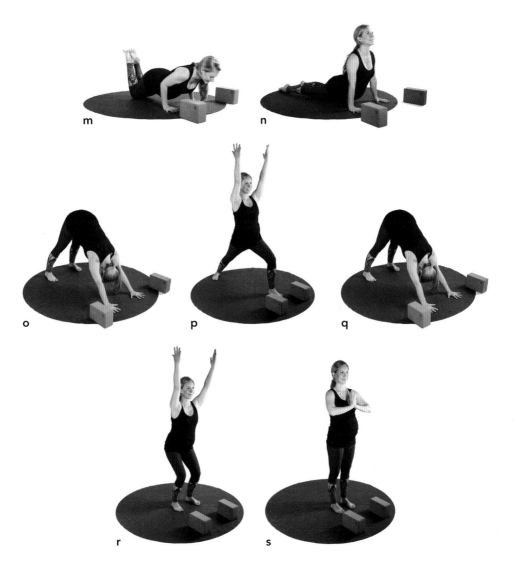

Half Sun Salutation and Sun Salutation A were described in chapter 4. Sun Salutation B offers you another sequence to help build strength. Choose the Salutation option that works best for you, which may change from day to day.

Benefits

This sequence warms the entire body; it's an effective warm-up for the upper body, lower body, and core.

Feeling

Inviting the feelings of warmth, radiance, and strength can help bring in the solar energy that the name of the sequence implies. Greet the possibilities of a new day, a new dawn, with the courage of a warrior. Warrior 1 is all about the feeling of rising up. Feel your strength as a mother rising up to help guide you throughout the journey of motherhood.

> continued

Sun Salutation B   *> continued*

Instruction

- Begin with your feet hip width apart, standing tall in Mountain Pose with your hands at your heart (see figure a).
- Inhale and sit into Chair Pose as you lift the arms to the sky, working toward having your arms parallel with your ears (see figure b).
- Exhale and come into a very gentle Forward Fold with your hands supported by the blocks (see figure c).
- Inhale and lift your torso halfway up so that it is parallel with the floor in a Half Forward Fold (see figure d). Feel the strength in your lower back.
- Exhale and step your feet back to Down Dog (see figure e). (We transition to Down Dog because it is kinder to the lower back than stepping back to Plank Pose.)
- Shift forward to Plank Pose and drop your knees to modify the pose (see figure f).
- Exhale and bend the elbows straight back to move into Modified Chaturanga Pose (see figure g).
- Inhale and either take a soft Up Dog with the belly off the floor and the knees on the floor (see figure h), or go straight to Unicorn and Rainbow.
- Exhale and return to Down Dog (see figure i). Stay in Down Dog for three deep breaths.
- Inhale and rise up to Warrior 1 on the right, floating your arms up to the sky and feeling the power in your stance (see figure j).
- Exhale and step back to Down Dog (see figure k).
- Shift forward to Plank Pose and drop your knees to modify the pose (see figure l).
- Exhale and bend the elbows straight back to move into Modified Chaturanga (see figure m).
- Inhale and either take a soft Up Dog with the belly off the floor and the knees on the floor (see figure n), or go straight to Unicorn and Rainbow.
- Exhale and return to Down Dog (see figure o). Stay in Down Dog for three deep breaths.
- Inhale and rise up to Warrior 1 on the left, floating your arms up to the sky and feeling the power in your stance (see figure p).
- Exhale and step back to Down Dog (see figure q).
- Slowly step your feet forward and sit into your Chair Pose with feet hip width apart (see figure r).
- Inhale and rise to standing with your hands at your heart (see figure s).

Adjustments

If there is any pulling in the abdomen whatsoever, omit the soft Up Dog and replace with Unicorn and Rainbow by dropping onto your knees. If you have been diagnosed with diastasis recti or are carrying multiples, it's OK to skip the vinyasa sequence of Plank, Modified Chaturanga, and Up Dog and replace it with Unicorn and Rainbow. If you would like additional padding under your knees for any part of the sequence, keep a folded blanket near the back half of your mat.

Puppy Pose

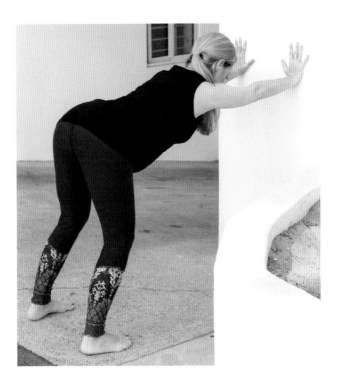

Benefits

This is a safe and easy way to stretch the lower back while supporting the weight of the upper body.

Feeling

Enjoy the feeling of traction in your spine. As you lengthen the crown of the head away from the tailbone, you can envision your spine as a ladder. With each breath cycle, sense, see, and feel a little bit more space between the rungs of the ladder.

Instruction

- Stand with your feet hip width apart and place your hands shoulder width apart on a wall slightly above the height of your hips.
- Slowly walk your feet back until your torso is parallel with the ground.
- Contract the muscles in your thighs and lengthen your tailbone back as you reach the crown of your head forward (see figure).

Adjustments

If you feel as though your knees are splaying out in this pose, consider placing a block between your thighs. You can turn the block to the width that allows you to leave a comfortable space between your thighs, and gently engage your inner thighs to help with proper alignment and stability in the pose.

Clock Squat

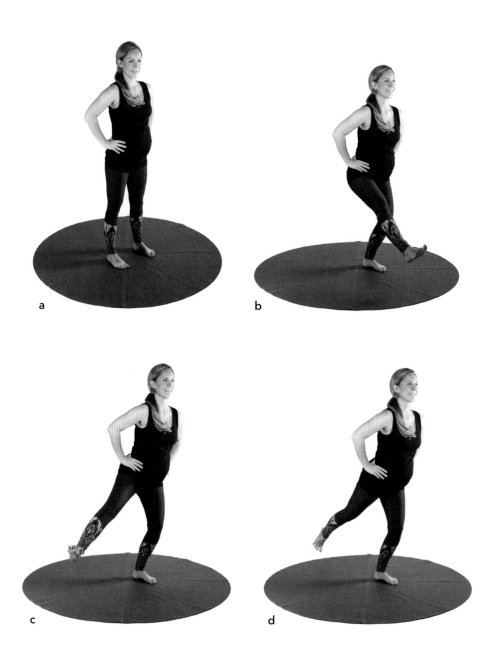

Benefits

This pose strengthens the hips and thighs and can help to build strength in the core stabilizers (glutes, quads, hamstrings, abductors, inner thighs, abs, lower back, obliques, and TVA).

Feeling

Imagine yourself standing on the face of a clock (see figure a). Remember that the standing foot is always pointed to twelve o'clock, so you are changing the time with the lifted foot.

Instruction

- Begin standing on your left leg with your right leg reaching out in front of you (as though the right leg were the hand of a clock pointing to twelve o'clock), hovering a few inches above the floor. Make sure your hips are parallel and your core is engaged. Keep your hands at your hips and stand up tall through the upper body. Bend your left knee as you inhale (see figure b), and then exhale and return to standing, still keeping the right leg above the floor.
- Now take your right leg out to the side (as though you were pointing it to three o'clock). Bend the left knee as you inhale (see figure c), and come back up to a straight leg as you exhale.
- Now take the right leg straight back (as though you were pointing to six o'clock). Repeat the sequence of bending the standing knee on the inhale (see figure d) and rising to a straight leg on the exhale.
- Finally, take the right leg across and back behind your standing leg (as though the right leg were pointing to eight o'clock), as in a curtsy, as you bend the standing leg on the inhale, and once again rise to straighten the leg on the exhale.
- Change sides and repeat the sequence standing on the right leg and bringing the left leg to twelve, nine, six, and four o'clock.

Adjustments

If you feel as though your balance is a little bit off, it is recommended that you place one of your hands on a stable surface, such as the bar on the side of a treadmill or the back of a sturdy chair. This will allow you to maintain your balance throughout the exercise.

Dancing Warrior

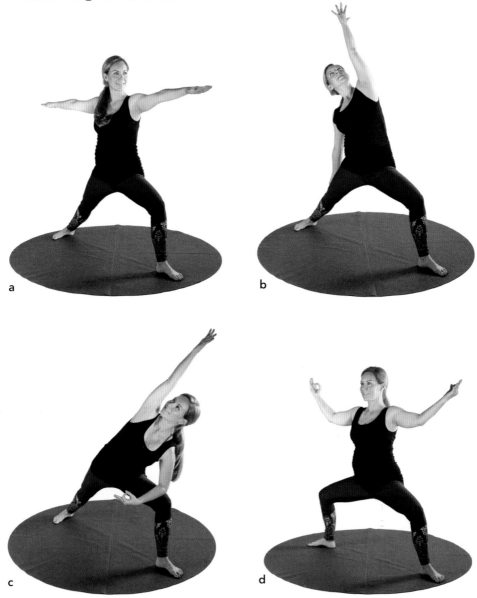

Benefits

This pose helps warm the entire body and cultivate strength in the lower body (quads, hamstrings, abductors, inner thighs) as you reach through a full range of motion in the upper body (flexibility training in the glenohumeral joints). The core stabilizers (TVA, abs, and lower back) are also active in the sequence.

Feeling

The feeling is that of rising up in Warrior 1 (or Crescent Lunge), expanding your energy and power in Warrior 2, feeling a sense of the exalted power in Reverse Warrior, and extending your power in Extended Side Angle. Feel the mama bear protective energy create a beautiful sacred space in your belly for your baby to grow and thrive. Surround this sacred space with the strength of your love, the strength of a mother.

Instruction

- Begin in Warrior 1 or Crescent Lunge with the left leg forward (this is a matter of preference; both are strong lunges, and both are correct) with your arms alongside your ears.
- Open to Warrior 2 on the exhalation and reach your arms out to the sides of the room. Bend the front knee and keep the back leg straight, with the back foot turned out slightly (see figure a).
- As you inhale, float the left arm up and back as you bring your right hand to your hip or thigh, stretching the left side of your torso in Reverse Warrior (see figure b).
- Exhale and reach the right arm alongside your ear in Extended Side Angle as you place your left forearm on your front thigh (see figure c) or your right hand on the floor or the block.
- Take a moment in Goddess Pose before you change sides (see figure d).
- Repeat the sequence on the left side.

Adjustments

If you are feeling as though you need a little extra support under your pelvis, you can enjoy this sequence on a chair. The last three poses of the sequence work better on a chair than the first one does, so it is best to begin with Warrior 2. Straddle the seat of a folding chair and bend your right knee to a 90 degree angle as you straighten the back leg and open your arms out to the sides at shoulder level. Breathe into Warrior 2 and feel the strength in your arms as you expand your energy to the front and the back. Flow into Reverse Warrior on your inhale and into Extended Side Angle on the exhale. Take a moment in a wide plié (Goddess Pose) on the chair before you change sides.

Goddess Pose

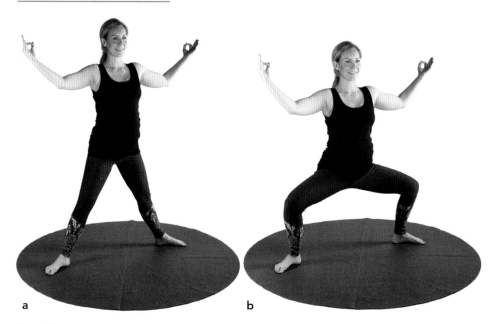

a   b

Benefits

This pose strengthens the lower body with particular emphasis on the inner thigh and, like the Clock Squats, can help build strength in the core stabilizers (glutes, quads, hamstrings, abductors, inner thighs, abs, lower back, obliques, and TVA).

Feeling

If you are or were a ballerina at any time in your life, remember the feeling of grace that this movement has as your powerful legs carry you up and down. If you are not a dancer, think of the beautiful quiet strength that ballerinas and ice skaters have. The movement looks easy and beautiful on the outside, and that is a direct result of the power and strength on the inside.

Instruction

- Begin standing with your feet a little bit wider than your shoulders.
- Let your hips rotate outward so that your feet are turned out to a 45 degree angle and your knees face the second toe of each foot (see figure a).
- Keep your spine erect and gaze forward as you inhale and bend your knees toward a 90 degree angle, keeping your knees turned out (see figure b).
- Exhale as you press to standing, emphasizing the strength in the inner thigh as it helps you drive back up to standing. Your abs will be lightly engaged in the movement to provide you with additional core stabilization.

Adjustments

If there is any challenge in keeping the upper body upright, you can place your hands on the back of a chair and use it as a ballet bar. This can help you find your balance as the weight of your growing belly and breasts begins to pull your torso forward. Note that the bottom of the plié is the same as what is called Goddess Pose in yoga.

Bent-Over One-Arm Row

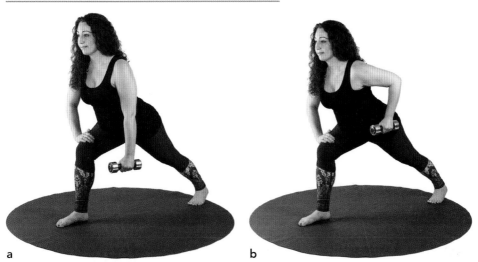

a   b

Benefits

This exercise strengthens the muscles of the rhomboids, also known as the posture muscles.

Feeling

Powerful posture muscles can help you to stand upright like a queen. As you draw your elbow back, feel the strength in the rhomboids and envision the power in the back of your body. During pregnancy, it is easy to focus on what is happening in the front of the body. This is totally normal since there is a beautiful baby growing in your belly. Remember to cultivate strength in your back to help balance and support all the miraculous changes that are happening in the front of your body.

Instruction

- Stand with your left hand holding a dumbbell and your right hand on your right quadricep or a stability ball (see figure a) or your forearm on a chair or a bench (if you are using a chair or bench, you can put your right knee on it).
- Hinge at the hips and keep your spine long and your gaze forward and down.
- Keep your palm facing in toward your torso as you exhale and pull your left shoulder blade in toward your spine as you pull the elbow back and up (see figure b). Keep the weight close to your body and feel the posture muscles contract at the top of the movement.
- Inhale and let the arm return to the straight starting position.
- Repeat 10 to 12 times, and then change sides.

Adjustments

This exercise can be performed with a small hand-held weight or a heavy but slim water bottle. Choose a weight that is challenging enough to build strength but not so hard that you cannot draw your shoulder blades in toward your spine. Bent-Over One-Arm Rows can be done with support from a chair, a stability ball, a couch, or a weight training bench. It can also be beneficial to begin with your nondominant side. For example, if you are right-handed, start with your left hand so that you can be sure to do the same number of repetitions on each side.

Standing Hip Abduction

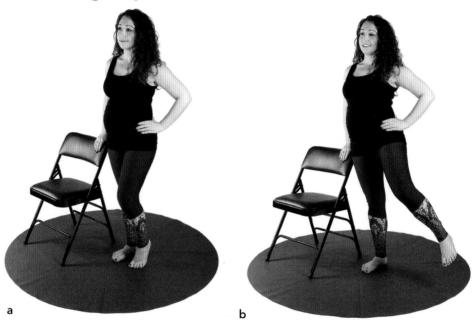

a   b

Benefits

This exercise helps strengthen the outer thighs and hips and the core.

Feeling

The outer thigh and hip muscles do not get a lot of work in daily life because they are responsible for movement from side to side. Unless you play tennis or ski, these muscles might be a little sluggish. Imagine these muscles lighting up and firing up each time you lift your leg. These muscles help to stabilize your legs and are a great source of power and strength in the lower body.

Instruction

- Stand next to a chair with your feet pointed straight ahead and your right hand at the top edge of the chair so that you have a makeshift ballet bar (see figure a).
- Keep your core muscles engaged and your right leg straight and strong as you slowly lift the left leg to the side and away from the midline into a comfortable stretch of the inner thigh (see figure b). The toes of your left foot will point straight ahead and you will feel the muscles in your outer hip and thigh contract at the top of the movement. When you are doing this correctly, it is completely normal to feel the muscles of your standing leg contract as well.
- Repeat 10 to 12 times; try to do so without touching the floor. Each time you lift your leg, exhale on the way up and challenge yourself to lift the leg just an inch or two higher each time.
- Repeat on the other side.

Adjustments

For more of a challenge, you can do this exercise without holding onto a chair. If you choose to do that, make sure there is a generous bend in the standing leg, especially during the second trimester. The bend in the standing leg will help you distribute your weight in such a way that you will not feel pulled forward.

Standing Push-Up

Benefits

This exercise helps strengthen the chest, shoulders, and arms.

Feeling

Think about strongly pushing the wall away from you. Imagine that you are a superhero (because you are!), and feel the strength in your chest and arms as you push the wall away from you. This action is very similar to many of the actions of Wonder Woman. She has great upper body strength to push away what could cause harm.

Instruction

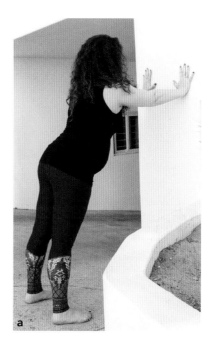

- Stand with your hands on a wall at the height of your shoulders and slowly walk your feet back a few inches until you can create a diagonal line with the length of your body (see figure a). Be aware that you are not allowing your hips to pull very far back (as in Puppy Pose) nor are you dropping into an overly swayed back with the lower back collapsing.
- On your inhalation, bend your elbows out to the sides of the room until your face comes close to the wall (see figure b).
- On the exhalation, use the strength of your arms to push away from the wall. Feel your chest muscles working in toward the midline at the top of the movement.

Adjustments

This is a traditional push-up turned on its side so that there is no risk of having your belly on the floor. If you feel as though you need a little bit more of a challenge, perform the push-up with your hands on a weight bench. With either variation, remember that if you ever feel like you do not have control of the movement, simply step one foot forward to balance your body.

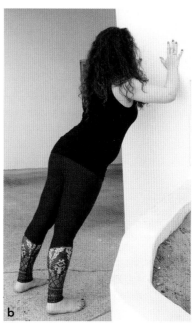

Lower Back and Hip Stretch

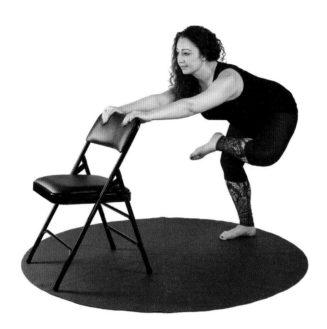

Benefits

This pose stretches the lower back and the outer hip of the lifted or crossed leg.

Feeling

This pose has a few different names. Some people call it Thread-the-Needle when it is practiced seated or lying down; others call it a Figure 4 Stretch because the legs are in the configuration of the number 4. The name Figure 4 is most applicable to the standing variation because the pose is completely angular, without any curved edges. Everything is elongated: the spine, the arms, and the back of the standing leg. Try to find the feeling of creating strong angles in this pose to create strong alignment.

Instruction

- Stand with your arms straight and your hands on a stable surface that you can hold onto, such as a kitchen or bathroom counter, a chair back, or the side bar of a treadmill.
- Cross your left ankle on top of your right thigh and gently sit your hips back as you bend your right knee (see figure).
- Elongate your spine and feel that your head is an extension of your spine so that you can maintain the correct alignment in the back of your body. Breathe into this powerful stretch and feel the muscles begin to release.
- You are stretching large muscle groups, so enjoy the stretch for as long as you like, up to 90 seconds, and then change sides.

Adjustments

This stretch is effective for releasing tensions in your lower back and is also fantastic for new moms who might have lower back pain as a result of picking up heavy gear (car seats, strollers, etc.), and then twisting while trying to turn and load gear into a car or truck. Remember that this stretch is portable, so you can enjoy it virtually anywhere at any time. If you feel pain creeping up in your lower back, hip, or both, consider using a street sign pole or a parking meter as your support and enjoy the stretch right before or after you drive your vehicle.

Putting It All Together

To create a balanced exercise plan for the second trimester, try to include daily meditation and 10 minutes of walking each morning and evening. Then, every other day, choose one of the following two workouts.

BE BRAVE: SECOND TRIMESTER HYBRID YOGA AND STRENGTH TRAINING PRACTICE

During the second trimester, your body expands to make space for your beautiful baby. As your belly begins to pull forward, it is important to keep the back of your body very stable and strong, both to support your posture and to avoid pain. It is common for the midback muscles to get sore as your breasts grow and pull your shoulders forward. Keeping the midback muscles strong will help you maintain good posture and not slump forward. Also, the lower back can get a little bit sensitive and even unstable at the SI joint. Low back pain is a common complaint during this time. This practice is designed to keep you standing tall like a queen, with a stable lower back that is supported from the inside out. Note that resistance tubing and water bottles or weights are needed for this practice.

Exercise	Page	Focus	Reps/Time
Standing meditation in Mountain Pose	45	Finding center	1 minute of full, slow, deep breathing; can be diaphragmatic breathing if comfortable, or simply breathe naturally and fully
Half Sun Salutation	48	Shoulders, core strength, flexibility	3 rounds; remember that each movement corresponds to an inhalation or exhalation
Clock Squats	84	Thighs, quads, glutes, core	4 reps on the right, 4 reps on the left; repeat 2 times
Goddess Pose	88	Inner thighs, core stabilizers	10-12 reps; repeat 2 times
Dancing Warrior	86	Lower body stability	2 times on each side using light (1-3 -lb) weights or full water bottles

Exercise		Page	Focus	Reps/Time
Superset: Do each exercise one time through and then repeat the entire sequence	Bent-Over One-Arm Row	89	Upper and middle back	12-15 reps on each side using light (1-3 -lb) weights or full water bottles; repeat 2 times
	Standing Hip Abduction	90	Outer thigh and hip	12-15 reps each side; repeat 2 times
	Standing push-up	91	Chest, upper arms, shoulders (pectorals, triceps, deltoids)	10-12 reps; repeat 2 times
Open-door chest stretch		72	Chest (pectorals)	5-10 deep breaths
Lower back and hip stretch		92	Lower back and outer hip	5-10 deep breaths on each side
Seated meditation in Easy Pose		41	Relaxes entire body	1-2 minutes or as long as your body needs to rest; sit on cushion if needed

RISE AND SHINE: ENERGIZING SECOND TRIMESTER PRACTICE

Your body is probably feeling stronger than it did during the first trimester. The fatigue is lifting and you have the opportunity to work with this return of energy to rise and shine. You can enjoy this particular practice at any time of day, but the energy is definitely focused on the feeling of sunshine. Yogis have many different variations of saying hello to the new day; these are called Sun Salutations. Take the time to invite a clear vision of warmth and radiance, like the rays of the sun, as you feel yourself rise and shine. Note that yoga blocks and a yoga bolster (or pillow) are needed for this practice.

Exercise	Page	Focus	Reps/Time
Child's Pose	59	Stretches lower back and hips, invites ease	9 slow, deep, centering breaths focusing on the inhalation and the exhalation being equal in length
Unicorn and Rainbow Pose	42	Warms the abs, TVA, and lower back	3 rounds inhaling as you gaze up, exhaling as you round the spine; you may place padding under the knees if you wish
Down Dog Pose	44	Lower back, hamstrings, calves	5 slow, deep breaths
Puppy Pose	83	Lower back, thighs	5 deep breaths
Half Sun Salutation	48	Shoulders, core strength, flexibility	3 rounds; remember that each movement corresponds to an inhalation or exhalation
Sun Salutation B	80	Entire body	1-3 rounds; remember that each movement corresponds to an inhalation or exhalation

Exercise	Page	Focus	Reps/Time
Tree Pose	55	Strengthens the stabilizers of the standing leg and external rotators of the lifted leg's hip	5-9 deep breaths on each side
Garland Pose	63	Hips and ankles	9 deep breaths
Pigeon Pose	56	Outer hip, lower back	9 deep breaths on each side
IT Band Twist	57	IT band	3 deep breaths on each side
Upward-Facing Table Pose	58	Lower back, shoulder strength	3 deep breaths
Deep Relaxation Pose	66	Entire body	3-5 minutes
Seated meditation in Easy Pose	41	Relaxes entire body	1-3 minutes; sit on cushion if needed

*M*ommy Move

Managing the Wave That Keeps on Waving

During pregnancy you will see your belly and breasts grow, especially in the second and third trimesters. Some of this weight is your baby, the placenta, and additional blood volume in your body. It is normal to also store some extra fat in your arms. In addition to having a sensible, nutritious eating plan and walking plan, make sure that you also take the time to enjoy some light weight training. Your upper body strength will be especially important when you are carrying your little one in your arms several hours a day.

The triceps are the muscles in the back of the upper arm. Women have many names for this area, the funniest one being *the wave that keeps on waving*. If you notice that your triceps are not toned and that they seem to wiggle and jiggle when you are waving hello to someone, now is a great time to get them in shape. As the name implies, there are three parts to this muscle group. The prefix *tri* means three and *cep* comes from the Latin word for head, indicating that the muscle has three heads; the lateral, the medial, and the long. In order to train this muscle group effectively, think about using your arm strength when the arms are stretched overhead as in Warrior 1, when they are pushing down in front of you as in a triceps pushdown or Modified Chaturanga, and when they are extending straight while slightly behind your hips as in a triceps dip or Upward-Facing Table. Targeting all three heads will help tone your triceps.

*I*nformation No One Tells You

Nasal Congestion

You may experience a lot of nasal congestion during the second trimester. There's conflicting information about the safety of decongestants and allergy medicines. Unless you have your ob/gyn's specific clearance or a prescription for nasal congestion medication, you will probably want to find a natural alternative for over-the-counter drugs. Here are some natural ways to help clear up nasal congestion.

- *Use a humidifier.* Increased moisture in the air helps prevent nasal dryness.
- *Try a neti pot.* This helps keep your nasal passages moist and clear; make sure to follow the directions and use only with distilled water.
- *Diffuse eucalyptus.* The scent of eucalyptus oil in the air can help open you up.
- *Chew gum.* Chewing mint-flavored gum can help moisturize your mouth and clear your sinuses.
- *Drink water.* Much like swallowing relieves pressure when you are on a plane, drinking water will encourage you to swallow more and help dissipate the sinus pressure.

Love-Your-Baby Visualization

Feeling Your Baby's Love for You

Sitting in Easy Pose with your back supported against a wall, take a moment to close your eyes and enjoy a deep, centering breath. Feel your sit bones pressing into the earth and the crown of your head rising up toward the sky. The energy of the lower body is grounded, providing a strong foundation upon which you can feel the energy of the upper body rising, like a tree growing upward. At the junction of these two energies, the grounding energy and the rising energy, is your baby. Connect to the feelings of love that you have for your little one. Feel the heart center energy being awakened in a new way as you prepare to meet one of the loves of your life in a few short months.

Now take a moment to consider that out of all of the billions of possibilities in the universe, you and your baby have come together. The Eastern traditions teach that the baby chooses its mother and that the souls already know each other. If this concept is in alignment with your own philosophy, then it will feel natural. If it is not in alignment with your beliefs, feel free to leave it off to the side. Either way, it is possible to feel the love that your baby has for you already. As you breathe into the sense of love that you have for your baby, allow yourself to become the receiver of your baby's communication toward you. You have the baby's favorite voice, favorite smell, favorite everything… you are mommy and you are deeply loved. When you feel a sense of completion with this meditation, speak the words *I love you, too* aloud so that your baby can hear and feel the vibration of love that emanates from within you, and as an outside sound of compassion.

Fun Foods

Spinach is high in folic acid, which is important for baby's brain development. Folic acid helps prevent neural tube defects (NTDs), which are serious birth defects of the spinal cord (e.g., spina bifida) and the brain (e.g., anencephaly). Spinach salad is a great form of taking in folic acid, and you can add protein and fat to balance your meal. This recipe is vegan and vegetarian friendly. If you would like more protein in this salad, you can add tofu or another protein source of your choice.

Spinach and Citrus Salad

    8 ounces baby spinach leaves
    1 large navel orange, peeled and segmented
    2 small avocados, sliced
    1/2 cup almonds
    Oil
    Vinegar
    Salt and pepper

Mix the ingredients together and add oil, vinegar, salt, and pepper to taste.
You can also make your own vinaigrette with those four ingredients plus some of the zest from the orange.
Yield: *2 large servings*

During pregnancy, bed rest is sometimes necessary. Although it can be challenging to stay in bed, you can still cultivate your warrior mama spirit by staying strong mentally and emotionally. Prescribed by health care practitioners for varying reasons, bed rest is a way of helping to bring more blood flow to the placenta; your doctor will let you know how long this time will last. Sometimes bed rest is prescribed for a few days, other times for a few weeks, or (rarely) for a few months. Varying levels of activity will be prescribed during this time. Some women are OK to continue walking around the house as long as they don't lift heavy objects. Other women are advised to stay in bed in an upright or reclined position, only leaving the bed to use the shower or the toilet. Your doctor will let you know what the recommendations are for you during pregnancy. Please note that bed rest is different from pelvic rest. For pelvic rest, there is a separate list of guidelines, which usually include avoiding the use of tampons and avoiding activities such as sex, repetitive squatting, and lower body training.

Bed rest can be challenging physically, mentally, and emotionally. Physically, there is increased risk of blood clots, poor circulation to your extremities (hands and feet), and additional weight gain or weight loss. Mentally, you may experience boredom, anxiety (worrying about all of the things you "should" be doing), or both. Emotionally, bed rest can be tough, especially for moms who have other children. Not being able to take your toddler to school can cause stress not just because you miss them, but also because there is the new burden of finding reliable child care. With so much happening in your mind, body, and heart, it can be beneficial to have a regular, sustainable, and above all *safe* practice that can help you move your body very gently as well as combat stress and anxiety. I designed the following practice for the journal *Fit Pregnancy* to help combat boredom, find a deep sense of center and peace, keep the blood moving to your extremities, and stay connected to your body and your baby.

1. *Breathe deeply.* Close your eyes and slow down your breath and your thoughts. Breathe deeply through the nose, sensing a kind of whispery feeling in the back of the throat. (If that's uncomfortable, you can breathe through the mouth.) Expand the time each breath takes; if you're used to breathing in for three seconds and out for two, try to make both your inhale and exhale closer to four seconds to calm and relax your body and mind.

2. *Visualize your baby.* Imagine baby's head pointed down toward your pelvis, and the back to your belly. Spend a few moments sending love, blessings, laughter, and peace to your little one.

3. *Take a gentle backbend.* Sit upright, stretch forward slightly, and place your hands 6 to 12 inches behind you on the bed. Open your chest, lift your heart and, if it feels okay, let your head dip back slightly for a breath or two. This easy backbend stretches the front of your body and your tired shoulders.

4. *Engage your shoulders.* Try weight-free Is, Ys and Ts: sit up in bed and lift your arms directly overhead for one breath (like a capital I), then out to the upper corners of the room (like a capital Y), then straight out to the sides (like a capital T). Perform three sets to encourage movement and blood flow to your upper body.

5. *Squeeze a ball.* Use your hands to squeeze a stress ball (or other small, pliable ball), breathing deeply as you squeeze. Imagine any stress, anxiety, or frustration moving out of your body and into the ball as you squeeze; just don't hold your breath.

6. *Try a supported stretch.* Arrange three pillows on your bed in a T shape, one horizontally at the top (for your head) and two underneath it vertically (for your spine). Lie back on the pillows, bend your knees, allowing them to open out to the sides. If your legs feel tight, place pillows under your outer thighs and knees. Relax and enjoy the stretch for at least one minute.

Originally published in *Fit Pregnancy*® magazine. All rights reserved.

6

Third Trimester: Prepare to Push

Welcome to the third trimester, mama! Your body is in full bloom with your growing baby, and you might be giggling about how only a few months ago you wondered *When will I start showing?* The added weight of your baby inside your body is supported by the pelvic floor muscles. These muscles are like a hammock that can stretch a bit with the added weight of your baby. These are also the muscles that will help you to push if you are having a vaginal delivery. Whether you have a vaginal delivery or a C-section, it is important to focus on these muscles so that you can carry the weight of your baby comfortably. Training your pelvic floor now can also help prepare you for recovery after you give birth.

Your Body in the Third Trimester

The third trimester is the home stretch of your pregnancy! At or around the 28th week of pregnancy, your baby will weigh approximately two and a half pounds and will be about the size of a small sweet potato and as long as a bok choy. When it is born, your baby will most likely weigh somewhere between 6 and 10 pounds, but Mother Nature has put some amazing systems in place to set you and your baby up for success. Pelvic floor muscles help to hold the weight of your baby throughout pregnancy and also help you push when it is time for labor and delivery.

The term *pelvic floor* has just started to reach the mainstream media so you will start to see pelvic floor exercises in fitness and yoga magazines. Yogis have known the power of the pelvic floor for centuries. In the practice of yoga, engaging your pelvic floor strength is known as *mula bandha,* which means *root lock.* You may recognize the term *mula* from chapter 3. The root chakra is called *muladhara.* But don't worry; you don't need to study Sanskrit to learn about the pelvic floor. Just keep in mind that in yoga the pelvic floor is referred to as the *root.*

The ancient yogis saw the spine as the central channel, or the tree of life. Trees have roots, and this metaphorical tree, the spine, has two types of roots: energetic and physical. The energetic root is the root chakra, which gives the feeling of grounding and connecting to Mother Earth. (Think of how, when you are jogging or dancing, you really feel present in your whole body.) The physical root is represented by the muscles of the perineum. By locating these muscles and learning to relax and softly contract them, you can feel a gentle lift. This gentle lift is the root lock that yogis refer to.

My approach to health, fitness, and pregnancy is to learn from both Eastern and Western traditions and use the best of both worlds to empower you as a mother. As a yoga teacher, I know that connecting to the energy of the root lock can help strengthen the perineal muscles. As an exercise science practitioner, I know that the pelvic floor works in harmony with your abdominal muscles. The abdominal muscles interdigitate (interlace, or interlock) with the pelvic floor muscles. If you interlace your fingers, you will see how they connect and weave together. Similarly, the lower belly muscles connect to your pelvic floor muscles, working together to help you carry the weight of your baby and eventually to give birth. Keeping these muscles strong through yoga and fitness exercises will set you up for success throughout your pregnancy, labor and delivery, and recovery.

A woman's pelvis is structurally a bit different from a man's because our bodies are built to allow for childbirth. The pelvic floor is a group of muscles and ligaments that form a floor that supports the uterus, bladder, and rectum. It is shaped like a diamond (see figure 6.1). The front of the diamond is called the urogenital space, through which your baby will be born if you have a vaginal delivery. The back of the diamond, which includes the rectum, is called the rectal space. There are muscles that reach from the front of the diamond to the back of the diamond, which is to say from your pubic bone to your tailbone. There are also muscles that reach from side to side.

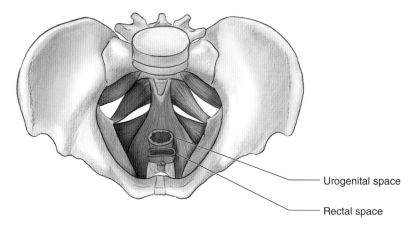

Urogenital space

Rectal space

Figure 6.1 The front and the back of the pelvic floor diamond.

Keen on Kegels

You might have been advised by your doctor or your trainer to do Kegel exercises. (They are named for Dr. Arnold Kegel who, in 1948, published his work on toning the pelvic floor muscles.) Kegel exercises involve repeatedly contracting and relaxing your pelvic floor muscles. These exercises can help strengthen the pelvic floor, which in turn helps prevent bladder leakage. Here is how to get started with Kegel exercises.

Identify the Correct Muscles

To correctly perform Kegels, you will need to locate the PC (pubococcygeal muscles). You can do this by trying to pause the flow of urine midstream. If you can pause when you pee, then you have found the right muscles. (Make sure not to pause when urinating as a regular technique because it can lead to urinary tract infection.)

Refine the Technique

Contract your pelvic floor muscles, hold the contraction for five seconds, and then relax for five seconds. Try it four or five times in a row. Work up to keeping the muscles contracted for 10 seconds at a time and relaxing for 10 seconds between contractions. Note that it is common to squeeze your abdominal muscles and gluteal muscles when trying to work your pelvic floor. Try to relax your tummy and your bottom (glutes), and make sure that you are not holding your breath.

Exercise in the Third Trimester

Not so long ago, women were told to relax and put their feet up during the third trimester. Now that we know the many benefits of exercise for mommy and baby, it is important to indicate which exercises are safe and effective. Third trimester workouts and yoga practices incorporate a lot of what you have learned in the first and second trimesters, with special attention and focus on your pelvic floor muscles.

We know that pelvic floor training can be beneficial for expecting moms because it can help support the extra weight of pregnancy, shorten the second stage of labor, and (because of increased circulation) increase the rate of healing after baby is born. Since the groundbreaking work of Dr. Kegel in the 1940s there have been many advancements in the field of pelvic floor dysfunction, and physical therapists have developed new and varied techniques for strengthening your pelvic floor.

Many birth professionals recommend the use of a Swiss ball (or a birthing ball, as a doula or midwife might call it) to help your baby get into a good position for labor and delivery. (You can also use a Swiss ball during your pregnancy as a prop in many exercises and stretches.) The ball is an integral part of the Push It workout, which is designed to help you increase your pelvic floor strength to prepare for pushing during labor (see workout later in this chapter). Bear in mind that there are benefits to strengthening the pelvic floor muscles even when you know that you are going to have a C-section. The pelvic floor has to hold the weight not just of your organs but also of your baby throughout the pregnancy, so strong muscles in the pelvis offer support.

Finding Your Calm in the Third Trimester

The third trimester is often the time when moms- and dads-to-be install baby's car seat, pack the bag for the hospital, and daydream about becoming parents. This period can feel like hurry-up-and-wait; everything is being prepared, and the days feel at once long and as though there's not enough time to prepare. Anticipation, finding a comfortable position for sleeping, and perhaps a little bit of uncertainty about how your life will change can leave you feeling anxious and unsure. Here is a list of my favorite ways to help find a sense of calm (and better sleep) in the third trimester.

- *Meditate regularly.* Studies show that a regular meditation practice can help reduce anxiety and stress.
- *Walk regularly.* Walking can help improve your mood and reduce stress.
- *Eat a balanced diet.* Feelings of well-being are encouraged by enjoying a diet that provides complex carbohydrates, essential fats, amino acids, vitamins and minerals, and water.
- *Enjoy essential oils.* Consider purchasing an essential oil diffuser and diffuse your favorite calming scent, such as lavender, in your living room or bedroom.
- *Write in a journal.* Keeping a pregnancy journal can serve you with important information if you have a future pregnancy, as well as being of interest to your children as they grow up. Kids love to know if their favorite food now was the same as your food cravings during pregnancy!
- *Enjoy calming music.* You do not have to be a professional DJ to create your perfect playlist; many mixes and ideas are available online.
- *Relax in Legs-Up-the-Wall Pose.* This yoga pose, which you'll find later in this chapter, will help induce calmness and can also relieve swollen ankles.

Also, keeping these muscles strong can lead to faster recovery. The ball can also be used after you have had the baby to help you get back into shape and to gently bounce with your baby in your arms when he needs soothing.

Here's some information to help you understand how best to use a Swiss ball, and how to choose one that's right for you. In choosing a ball, first look for the size of ball that best fits your height (see table).

It's also important to look for a label

Exercise ball diameter	Your height
45 cm	5' and under
55 cm	5'1"-5'8"
65 cm	5'9"-6'2"
75 cm	6'3"-6'7"

on the box or website that you are purchasing from that says *anti-burst technology* to help ensure it's a safe piece of equipment to use throughout your pregnancy and beyond.

Yoga Poses and Exercises for the Third Trimester

The following poses are listed to increase your power for pushing during the third trimester, and there are cues for enjoying each pose throughout your pregnancy. Move slowly, breathe deeply, and enjoy your yoga practice.

Hip Circle

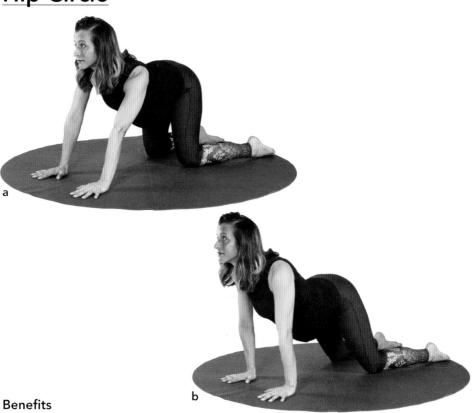

a

b

Benefits

This movement offers a dynamic stretch of the hips and lower back while also engaging the core.

Feeling

If you have ever made cookies at home, you know that little kids (and adults) often like to scrape some of the batter off the inside of the bowl with a spatula to enjoy every bit of sweetness. Imagine that your hips are the spatula and that you are trying to scoop your hips all the way around, all 360 degrees of the circle, to get every bit of sweetness; in this case the sweetness is a satisfying stretch for your lower back and hips.

Instruction

- Begin on all fours with your hands shoulder width apart and knees hip width apart.
- Gently circle your hips around in one direction while keeping a slight bend in your knees (see figures a and b).
- For the third trimester of pregnancy, perform the exercise slowly and enjoy several circles in one direction before you pause and change sides.

Adjustments

You can perform this exercise while sitting on a stability or birthing ball, especially as you get closer to labor and delivery. Move slowly and make sure you are working on a nonslip surface (not carpet), and that you are either wearing supportive athletic shoes or are barefoot with your feet on a sticky mat (most yoga mats have some grip or stickiness to them to keep you from slipping).

Standing Lateral Stretch

Benefits

This movement stretches the side body (latissimus dorsi, intercostals, obliques).

Feeling

The side of the body does not usually receive as much attention as the front and the back of the body. Enjoy the feeling of lengthening in the side body, and remember that the little muscles between your ribs help you to enjoy deep breathing. Imagine that you can breathe even deeper into the right lung as you bend to the left, and vice versa.

Instruction

- Stand with your feet hip width apart and sweep your arms overhead. Interlace your fingers and turn your palms to the sky.
- On an inhalation, lengthen through the spine and reach up actively through the arms.
- On your exhalation, reach over to the left as though you were bending up and over a large beach ball, so that you don't collapse the side of your body (see figure).
- Enjoy three to five deep breaths on the left and then return to center to reestablish balance. Then change sides.

Adjustments

If you are not able to bring your hands together because your shoulders are tight, you can choose to use a yoga strap or belt. Take the strap in your hands to fill the space between your hands. Gently walk your hands as close together as is comfortable before you enter the stretch.

Seated Thread-the-Needle Pose

Benefits

This pose stretches the outer thighs and hips and the glutes.

Feeling

The feeling is one of releasing and letting go. The outer hip and thigh are a large muscle group that can get tense without us even noticing it until we are in deep stretches. Take your time and breathe into the feeling of letting go of any tension that no longer serves you; imagine it releasing and relaxing more and more with each breath cycle.

Instruction

- Seated on a ball or chair, place your feet hip width apart.
- Cross your right ankle on top of your left thigh, and place your left hand against the sole of the right foot, with your right hand on top of your right thigh. Gently encourage the upward flexion (dorsiflexion) in your foot by pressing your left hand into your right foot. Press your right hand down actively onto the right thigh to encourage external rotation in the right hip.
- Now, elongate your spine and hinge forward at the hips, with the breastbone reaching forward and slightly down (see figure). Be aware that you are not rounding in the upper body, and that your head and neck are an extension of your long spine.
- Hold for 30 to 60 seconds, then switch to the other side.

Adjustments

If you would like a slightly more intense stretch, try this pose standing while keeping your hands safely holding onto a bar or the side of a treadmill. You can sit into the stretch and let your hips go back a little bit farther than they do in the seated variation. If you don't have a treadmill or a fixed bar you can hold onto, you can ask your spouse or significant other to let you hold onto their forearms as you sit back into the stretch.

Seated and Supported Wide-Legged Forward Fold

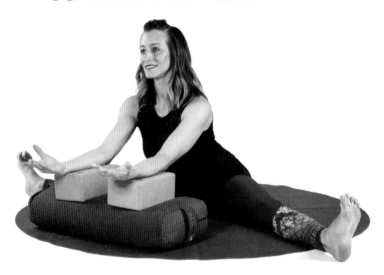

Benefits

This pose provides a deep stretch for the inner thighs and a gentle stretch for the lower back; it's also calming to the nervous system.

Feeling

Supported poses send a message to the nervous system that you are safe. Your body can settle into a deeper breath, and in this variation of Wide-Legged Forward Fold, there is a literal and figurative message to the brain that this vital organ is supported and safe. Breathe deeply into the feelings of support, safety, and comfort.

Instruction

- Begin seated on the floor with a folded blanket on the seat of a chair in front of you or with a bolster on the floor with blocks on top of it.
- Open your legs into a wide straddle position around the legs of the chair or around the bolster. Feel your sit bones pressing down into the floor and your knees and toes facing the sky.
- Lengthen through your spine on an inhalation, and on an exhalation, hinge at your hips and gently fold forward into a supported forward bend (see figure). You can have your forearms resting on the blocks or your arms folded on the chair or your hands reaching for the back of the chair; all are correct.

Adjustments

You can add another folded blanket under your sit bones if you would like additional cushion for your bottom. To move deeper into this pose, you can slide your forearms forward on the blocks or the chair forward slightly to get a deeper stretch. Please be cautious and remember that even if you are very flexible, it is important to leave space for your baby, and never to bear weight on your abdomen. Your belly should always hover above the floor.

Seated Head-to-Knee Pose (Open Variation)

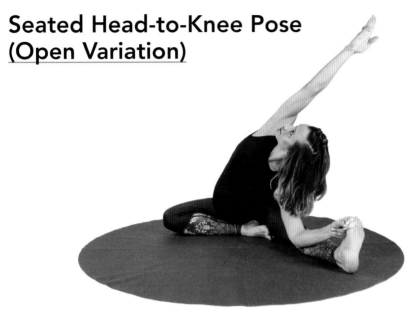

Benefits

This pose strengthens and stretches the legs, the rotators of the torso, and the muscles of the top arm.

Feeling

There is a distinct energy of spiral in this pose. Think of spiraling your heart center to the sky as your strong lower body remains grounded and provides a stable foundation. As in Extended Side Angle, there is a feeling of a strong and stable foundation, like the roots of a strong flower with the blossom turning toward the sun.

Instruction

- Begin seated on the floor. Bend your right knee and place the sole of the right foot against the inner left thigh.
- Bring your left hand to your left foot.
- Sweep the right arm alongside your ear and enjoy a deep side stretch in the right side of the waist (see figure). Make sure that you continue to lengthen the right side of the waist so that you are not collapsing the other side of the torso.
- If you are very flexible in the shoulders, you can reach the top hand all the way over your head. If there is any challenge in doing so, feel free to omit that option, and reach over to wherever you can.

Adjustments

Be aware that the variation described here is not the traditional pose, which is practiced with the heel of the left foot pressing into the pubic bone. Because this is contraindicated during pregnancy, we show it with the foot against the thigh for safety and comfort. If you need extra padding under your seat, use a folded blanket to give your hips some cushion.

Seated Goddess Pose

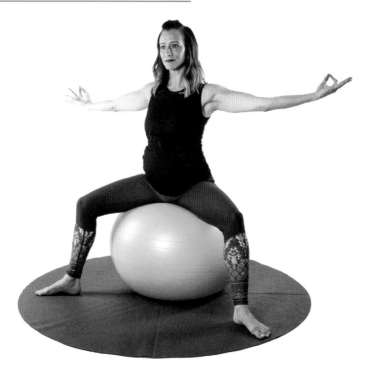

Benefits

This pose strengthens the lower body and core stabilizers and also offers light engagement of the upper body.

Feeling

Some teachers call this Temple Pose but it is more often referred to as Goddess Pose. Connect to the energy of your body as being full of grace, energy, and life, like a goddess.

Instruction

▎ Begin seated on the stability ball with your feet hip width apart on the floor. Slowly walk your feet out a little bit wider until they are about three or four feet apart and your hips and knees are externally rotated.

▎ Reach the arms out to the sides of the room at the height of your shoulders. You can choose to lift the hands gently and bring the thumb and pinkie together or simply let your palms face the sky in a gesture of receiving (see figure).

▎ Breathe into the pose and sustain the shape for several breaths.

Adjustments

This stretch can be done as an active stretch and an opportunity to work the strength of the pelvic floor at the end of each exhale, or it can be more of a passive stretch when performed while seated on a chair.

Seated Side-to-Side Rock

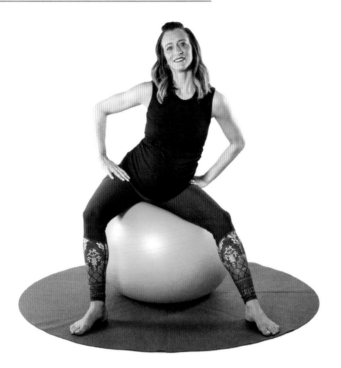

Benefits

This movement mobilizes the muscles of the pelvic floor.

Feeling

Experience the feeling of mobility in the hips as though you were a child simply enjoying playtime with a beach ball. This is a valid form of exercise that has distinct benefits for pelvic mobility, but it's also fun! Allow yourself to be playful and perhaps take a moment to think of all of the ways you can start to invite the spirit of play into your life. Soon you will be the mama of a little one who loves to play.

Instruction

- Sit on top of the stability ball with your feet a little bit wider than hip width apart. Sit up tall through your torso and put your hands on your hips or reach them directly in front of you at the height of your shoulders.
- Feel your sit bones gently pressing into the ball. Begin to shift your body weight more onto the left sit bone as you exhale (see figure). You will also feel a secondary contraction in your waist muscles (the obliques act as a synergist, an agent that increases effectiveness).
- Return to center, and then change sides. Enjoy several rounds of this exercise, and remember to breathe deeply and naturally. It can also be helpful to use what the yogis call a *dristi*, or focal point. Allow your gaze to rest gently on one point; this will help you keep your equilibrium.

Adjustments

If you feel unstable with this exercise, it's OK to place your ball at arm's length from the wall so you can tap the wall with your fingertips to reestablish your balance.

Seated Extended Side Angle Pose

Benefits

This pose strengthens and stretches the legs, the rotators of the torso, and the muscles of the top arm.

Feeling

In extended side angle, there is a beautiful feeling of turning your heart toward the sky. The Spanish word for sunflower is *girasol*, which means *to turn to the sun*. Let your heart turn to the sun like a beautiful sunflower.

Instruction

▌ Begin sitting on a stability ball with your feet about four feet apart and turn your left foot straight out to the left and your right foot slightly inward.

▌ Bend your left knee at a 90 degree angle while keeping the right leg straight and strong.

▌ Bring your left forearm to your left thigh and sweep your right arm alongside your ear as you bend your torso to the left (see figure).

▌ Feel the right side of your waist stay engaged and lengthened as much as you can comfortably while turning the right side of the torso to the sky.

▌ Enjoy several deep breaths as you continue to keep lengthening the right side of your torso.

▌ Come back up to the center, and then change sides.

Adjustments

This pose can also be practiced while standing on your mat or seated on a chair. Choose the variation based on your level of energy and the amount of support that you need under your pelvis on any given day. Also, note that you can place your bottom hand on top of a yoga block if there is space between your hand and the floor, although some practitioners choose to bend the bottom arm and use the front thigh as a shelf for the arm. Both variations (hand on block and forearm on leg) are correct. Think about choosing an option that feels most natural in your body and allows you to find a sense of spiral in the torso, as if your heart were spiraling up to the sky.

Wall Squat

Benefits

This move strengthens the hips, thighs, and core stabilizers.

Feeling

Feel a powerful sense of grounding through your feet as you enjoy this exercise. In the Eastern traditions, the legs correspond to the element of earth, so there is a natural sense of being grounded in the lower body. At the same time, feel the crown of the head rising toward the sky so that you have a sense of growing tall as a result of your supported, stable foundation.

Instruction

- Place a stability ball against the wall at the height of your hips, and turn your body away from the wall so that the ball rests gently above your tailbone as you step your feet hip width apart (see figure a). Your hands can rest on your hips or on top of your thighs if you prefer; both are correct.

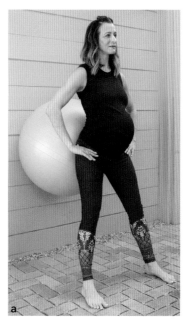

a

- Standing tall in your torso, inhale and squat down until your knees are at a 90 degree angle, making sure your knees are pointed straight ahead (see figure b). The ball will naturally roll up the length of your spine until it is just above the shoulder blades. Focus on the pelvic floor stretching in four directions at the bottom of the movement. Imagine that your pubic bone is moving forward, your tailbone is moving back slightly, and the sit bones are moving away from each other.
- As you exhale, straighten your legs and return to standing, gently engaging your glutes at the top of the movement. As you straighten your legs to stand up, feel a gentle lift in the pelvic floor, and imagine those same four bony landmarks (tailbone, pubic bone, sit bones) moving in toward the midline of the body. At the very top of the movement, you can also add a Kegel so there is a little extra contraction or lift of the pelvic floor.
- Repeat the exercise 12 to 15 times, remembering to coordinate your breath cycle with the movement.

Adjustments

If you have a tendency to let your knees either knock in or collapse out, place a yoga block between your inner thighs to maintain the proper alignment of your knees. If you would like an added challenge, you can add a Kegel exercise at the top of the squat. Feel the lift of the pelvic floor as you rise, emphasizing it as you straighten your legs.

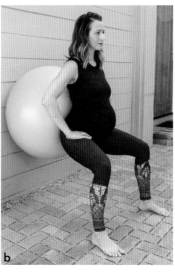

b

Kneeling Hip Abduction

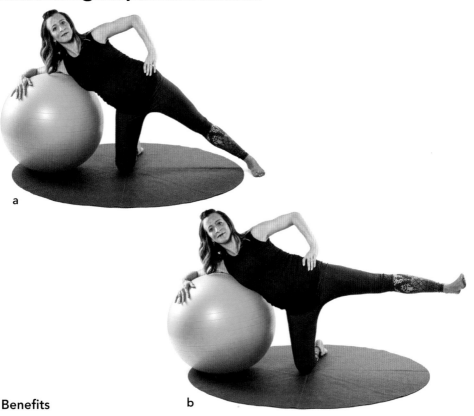

a

b

Benefits

This exercise strengthens the outer thighs and hips and stabilizes the core with the ball.

Feeling

This exercise can be a bit humbling; it's surprising how challenging it can be to simply lift your leg! Be patient with yourself and affirm that you are a strong and powerful mama and that this movement is simply another opportunity to overcome a challenge. Prove to yourself that you have a deep reservoir of strength you can draw from as needed.

Instruction

- Begin kneeling on the floor with the right side of your torso lying on the stability ball (see figure a). Place your right knee on the floor and your right forearm on the ball. Your left hand can rest on your left hip and your left leg will extend to straight.
- As you exhale, slowly lift your left leg until it is parallel with the floor (see figure b).
- As you inhale, let the leg come down until it almost touches the floor.
- Repeat 12 to 15 times, making sure that you are breathing deeply and comfortably. Then switch sides.

Adjustments

If you would like additional padding under your right knee, place a folded blanket there for cushion. You can tap the top foot to the floor any time you feel as though your balance is off. Take a moment with your foot on the floor to recalibrate and find your balance. Then continue the exercise when ready.

Seated Pelvic Roll

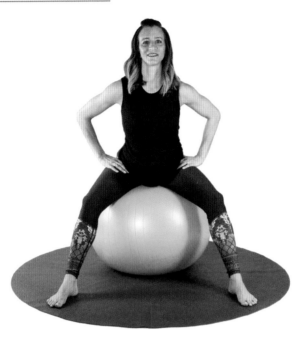

Benefits

This pose strengthens the muscles of the pelvic floor including the pubococcygeus (PC) muscles.

Feeling

Envision the muscles of the pelvic floor as a rose. With each inhalation the rose blossoms, and with each exhalation it returns to the more compact rosebud. Connect to the feeling of blossoming when you are working the pelvic floor; this will help you during labor and delivery.

Instruction

▌ Sit on top of the ball and take the time to roll a little bit from side to side to help locate your sit bones. Now roll a little forward and back until you can feel where your pubic joint (where the two pubic bones meet) and your tailbone are located.

▌ On your inhalation, imagine that the muscles running front to back from your pubic joint to your tailbone are stretching.

▌ On the exhalation, imagine the muscles running from front to back and the muscles running from side to side are moving in toward the midline (see figure). At the end of the exhale you can add a Kegel for an extra lift of the pelvic floor.

Adjustments

A yoga block is a great alternative to the stability ball for pelvic floor work. You can sit in yogi squat (*malasana*, aka Garland Pose) and allow the blocks to support your body weight. Sitting on blocks will give you a different feeling of support while at the same time stretching the calves. If your heels don't touch the floor while in your yogi squat, place a folded blanket under your heels to fill in the space between your heels and the floor.

Heart-Opening Stretch on Stability Ball

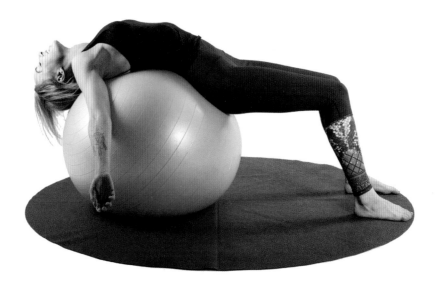

Benefits

This pose stretches the chest and shoulders.

Feeling

Enjoy the feeling of opening your arms wide as if to receive, and the light and energy of your heart center shine like the rays of the sun and expand from the inside outward. You are receiving the gift of motherhood; it can be sweet to reflect on the magnitude of this gift. On a purely physical level, this stretch feels very good after you have been working at the computer or in other positions where you round forward.

Instruction

- Sit on top of the stability ball with your feet hip width apart.
- Slowly walk your feet forward until your hips can easily come down off the ball. The ball will rest just above the waistband of your pants and will support your middle back, upper back, neck, and head.
- Open your arms wide and let your focus gently rest on the ceiling as you breathe into a deep yet passive stretch for the chest, shoulders, and arms (see figure). This stretch is passive in nature because, even though you are opening your arms wide, gravity will play a large part in opening the chest as your arms are gently drawn apart a bit farther, as if to give someone a big embrace.

Adjustments

On those days when you feel as though your balance is a bit off, place the ball up against a wall or a sofa for an added sense of stability and support.

Fortune-Teller

Benefits

This movement strengthens and mobilizes the pelvic floor muscles.

Feeling

The feeling of this movement is one of drawing everything in and gently up on the exhalation, and creating space on the inhalation. Or you can envision the pelvic floor muscles as a rose. On the inhalation, the flower is blossoming or opening, and on the exhalation it draws back in like a rosebud, in a continuous cycle. I call this the Fortune-Teller because it reminds me of the little folded-paper fortune-tellers we used to make at sleepaway camp to daydream about how many children we'd have and what kind of house we'd live in. The paper created four points that could move in toward the midline or away from it, much like the pelvic floor.

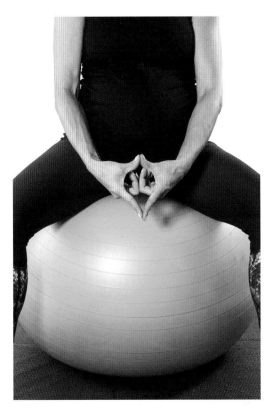

Instruction

- Sitting on a yoga block or stability ball, rock gently side to side and feel your sit bones. Imagine a band of muscle that stretches from side to side and connects these two bones.
- On your inhalation, feel and envision the sit bones moving away from each other as this muscle stretches.
- On the exhalation, feel and envision this muscle contracting toward the center and the sit bones moving closer to each other. Now rock front to back on the ball and locate your pubic joint and your tailbone. Again, imagine the band of muscle that stretches from front to back and connects these two bones.
- Now put it all together and as you inhale feel the sit bones moving away from each other and the pubic bones and the tailbone moving away from each other.
- On the exhalation, feel everything moving in toward the midline.

Legs-up-the-Wall Pose

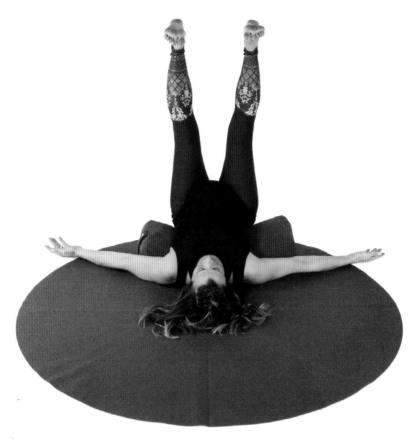

Benefits
This pose promotes a deep sense of relaxation and can help reduce edema (swelling) in the ankles.

Feeling
Another name for Legs-up-the-Wall Pose is Waterfall Pose. The feeling is that of energy cascading down your body like a soft waterfall of peace.

Instruction
- Place a bolster about three inches from the wall.
- Sit down on the bolster with your right shoulder and hip facing the wall.
- As you lie back onto your back, gently swivel your hips onto the bolster with your tailbone close to the wall, draped over the front edge of the bolster. Keep the legs hip width apart.
- Allow your arms to find a comfortable position out to the sides or with one hand on your heart and the other on your baby.

Adjustments
Use a lightly scented lavender eye pillow to promote rest.

Yoga and the Breech Position

Many expectant mothers ask if there's anything they can do about a breech baby. While there are different types of breech (complete, incomplete, frank, or transverse), the position means that the baby's bottom and feet, rather than the head, are facing the bottom of the uterus. If your baby is breech, it is recommended that you wait until you are 32 to 37 weeks pregnant to try to help the baby turn into the preferred birthing position, with the head down. Remember that babies have their own path. I recommend a four-step process for moms.

1. *Meditate.* Quiet your mind and go within. Ask your baby to turn head down, with its back to your belly.
2. *Invert.* Down Dog Pose can help babies to turn by creating space in the lower part of the uterus.
3. *Midwife.* Many midwives are skilled in the traditional Mexican rebozo technique, which can help the baby to turn.
4. *Chiropractor.* Highly skilled chiropractors who specialize in women's health can perform the Webster technique to get the baby into correct position.

If your baby does not turn, that is no reflection on you as a mother or as a woman. The most important thing in my opinion is a healthy mommy and a healthy baby. Your health care practitioner will provide you with the safe options available to you for bringing your baby into the world.

Putting It All Together

To create a balanced exercise plan for the third trimester, try to include daily meditation and 10 minutes of walking each morning and evening. Then, every other day choose one of the following two workouts.

PUSH IT: THIRD TRIMESTER PUSHING POWER PRACTICE

As you prepare for labor and delivery—in other words, as you get ready to push—it can be helpful to learn more about pelvic mobilization and feel the power of your pelvis. Note that this practice can be helpful even for mamas who know they are going to have a scheduled C-section. The weight of your baby is held by the hammocklike structure created by the pelvic floor muscles. These muscles benefit from gentle training not only during pregnancy but again for the recovery of muscular strength after you have your baby. It's also beneficial to stretch the shoulders and chest because the weight of your growing breasts will pull your shoulders forward. This workout will help you maintain good posture by gently stretching the upper body and strengthening your posture muscles. Note that you will need a small handheld weight (5 to 10 pounds), and a stability, or birthing, ball for this practice. Make sure the ball is the correct size for your height (see table earlier in this chapter), is filled properly with air, is labeled as anti-burst, and is safely sealed with the manufacturer-provided plastic pin.

Exercise	Page	Focus	Reps/Time
Seated Side-to-Side Rock	111	Pelvic floor and core stabilizers	10 rocks right to left; 2 sets
Seated Goddess Pose	110	Core stabilizers and gentle work for the legs	5-10 deep centering breaths
Wall Squats	113	Hips and thighs, core stabilizers	10-12 reps; 2 sets
Standing Lateral Stretch	106	Obliques	3-5 breaths each side; 2 sets

Exercise	Page	Focus	Reps/Time
Kneeling Hip Abduction	114	Outer thighs and hips	8-10 reps; 2 sets
Bent-Over One-Arm Row	89	Midback, or posture, muscles	8-10 reps each side; 2 sets
Fortune-Teller	117	Pelvic floor	1 minute
Heart-Opening Stretch on Stability Ball	116	Stretches the chest and shoulders	1 minute
Seated meditation in Easy Pose	41	Invites calm	3-5 minutes

TAKE IT EASY: THIRD TRIMESTER SUPPORTIVE PRACTICE

You are in the home stretch of pregnancy, and some days it feels good to take it easy. With the added weight of the third trimester, there will be some days when you might want to sit and have some extra support under the weight of your pelvis. This practice is designed to support your body weight. First, you are supported by your feet and standing in your strength. In the second part of the practice, you are supported by a chair, and in the third and final section, you are supported by Mother Earth. Move slowly and breathe into the energy of gentleness and ease. Note that a standard folding chair (if you are over 5'8", you might prefer a slightly taller chair) and a yoga bolster or a large pillow are needed for this practice.

Exercise	Page	Focus	Reps/Time
Standing meditation in Mountain Pose	45	Centering	1 minute
Unicorn and Rainbow Pose	42	Lower back and abdomen	5 rounds, inhaling as you gaze up, exhaling as you softly round
Hip Circle	105	Lower back and hips; pelvic mobilization	5 circles each side
Standing Lateral Stretch	106	Side body, including waist muscles	3 deep breaths right and left
Seated Goddess Pose	110	Opens and stretches the chest, front of the shoulders, and inner thighs	5-10 deep breaths

Exercise	Page	Focus	Reps/Time
Seated Extended Side Angle Pose	112	Side body including waist and back	5 deep breaths right and left
Seated Thread-the-Needle Pose	107	Outer thighs and hips	5-10 deep breaths right and left
Seated and Supported Wide-Legged Forward Fold	108	Lower back and inner thighs	5-10 deep breaths
Seated Head-to-Knee Pose (open variation)	109	Outer hip and thigh, side body	5-10 deep breaths right and left
Deep Relaxation Pose	66	Entire body	3-5 minutes

Mommy Move

The Knack

The Knack is the name of an exercise taught by physical therapists to help you avoid a pee sneeze. It is common for a bit of urine to leak when you sneeze during pregnancy and after. Strained, weak, and overstretched pelvic floor muscles can lead to light bladder leakage, or, as it is politely referred to these days, LBL. If you sometimes experience LBL, especially when sneezing, try this exercise.

- When you feel a sneeze or cough coming on, cross your legs.
- Activate your inner thigh muscles to contract along with the pelvic floor muscles.
- Actively contract and lift your pelvic floor muscles.

It is recommended to use the Knack at the onset of a natural sneeze or cough, but bear in mind that there are other, more effective ways of training the pelvic floor on a daily basis.

Information No One Tells You

Light Bladder Leakage

If you have LBL, you can of course use regular panty liners to protect your undergarments. Many feminine hygiene companies sell LBL pads, which are very similar to panty liners. Both work very well and can prevent embarrassing accidents. In addition to the Knack exercise, the pads will give you a backup source of protection. After labor and delivery, you can freeze the pads before you use them to help manage the lochia, or blood flow, that is normal after giving birth. By freezing the pads, you will have the added benefit of something cool to soothe damaged tissues as your body naturally repairs itself.

Love-Your-Baby Visualization

Looking Into Your Child's Eyes

Sitting in Easy Pose with a cushion under your hips and your back against a wall or a sofa, close your eyes. Allow your attention to turn inward, and slow your breath. Connect to the energy of your son or daughter. Breathe slowly and deeply and send your love to your little one. Now take a moment to imagine the first time that you hold your baby in your arms. You can start to imagine where this will take place, whether in the hospital or in your home. Take a moment to envision your face smiling as your doctor or midwife places your baby in your arms. Now imagine that you are looking at your beautiful baby with love in your heart and in your gaze. Envision your little one looking up at you. Imagine those little eyes opening to take in the world and to look at your face for the first time. For 40 weeks or so, your child has heard your voice, felt your love, and grown inside your body. Imagine the powerful loving gaze your baby will have at first sight of you. Allow yourself to feel the intensity of looking into the eyes of one of the loves of your life. Stay with the vision as long as feels natural. When you feel a sense of completion, gently flutter your eyes open, knowing that this vision will become a reality in a few short weeks or days.

Fun Foods

If you have ever eaten a snack that is very high in carbohydrate, such as a muffin, and felt a little sleepy about three hours later, chances are that your blood sugar spiked and then crashed. In order to stabilize your blood sugar, it is important to work toward a balanced diet including carbohydrate, protein, and fat at each meal. An easy way to do this is to add extra ingredients to something that is already part of your diet. For example, if you eat eggs (protein), you can add cheese (fat) and spinach (carbohydrate) to create a balanced meal. Here is one of my favorite recipes for cheesy eggs.

Spinach and Feta Omelet

Oil for the pan

1 clove garlic, diced

3 large eggs, lightly beaten

3 cups fresh spinach

1/3 cup crumbled feta cheese

Salt and pepper to taste

In a pan with a bit of oil, sauté the garlic for about 2 minutes. Add the spinach and cook until wilted (about 5 minutes). In a separate pan, cook the eggs on low heat in a little more oil until you can gently fold in the sides a bit to allow for more of the center to cook. When the eggs are almost fully cooked on top and fluffy, add the spinach, feta cheese, and garlic and cook for another minute. Slide the eggs out of the pan in one large piece and fold in half. Add salt and pepper to taste.
Yield: 1 serving

Happy Birth Day!

Today is the day you will meet one of the loves of your life. For many women the early stage of labor is rather mild and feels a bit like menstrual cramps. Others might feel lower back pain, and in about 15 percent of women the amniotic sac ruptures (aka the water breaking). Hollywood has given us some intense images of women standing in a checkout line with a sudden splash of water, needing to rush to the hospital, where they scream or swear at their spouse or partner. After about two minutes of movie time, a perfectly clean roundheaded baby emerges and the scene is over. This cinematic lore is not reality for the vast majority of women. Labor can be very different for different women; it can even be very different for the same woman experiencing her second or third pregnancy.

When you are preparing for labor and delivery, it can be helpful to have a birth plan. But remember that babies have their own plan, which can sometimes send our plans right out the window. Still, it's good to have your written birth plan in place so that the medical staff, midwife, and your family know what your intentions are for this experience. Just as we set a clear intention for our yoga practice, we can set a clear intention for the labor and delivery experience. Take a moment to reflect on what type of experience you would like to have. Do you want the room to be soft and relaxing, perhaps with classical music? Or do you want to play the song "Tootsie Roll" and *dance* your baby out? (Yes, a woman did this on YouTube, and it was fantastic.)

Whatever your plan is, try to surround yourself with people who are supportive of your vision. As a pre- and postnatal yoga teacher, I often encounter women who think I will tell them that the best way to have a baby is all natural, at home, with a midwife. This preconception arises from the stereotype that yoga teachers value all-natural over all else. But I'm a big fan of you having a birth experience in which you feel empowered, supported, and celebrated. As women and as moms, the last thing we need is to judge each other, or "should on each other." Whatever path lies ahead of you—vaginal delivery, C-section (scheduled or emergency), VBAC (*vee-back* for short: vaginal birth after C-section), natural delivery, medicated delivery, delivery with an ob/gyn, delivery with a midwife, delivery at home, delivery at the hospital—I recognize and honor your ability to choose what is right for you and your baby with the help of your team. From the perspective of someone in the fitness and yoga industry, I know firsthand the power of preparing your body, mind, and heart for any major life event, especially a physical event. In this chapter, we will explore some of the ways physical fitness and strength can translate into increased mental and emotional strength.

Mind–Body Connection

We have all heard of the power of the mind–body connection. When your body and your mind work together, it's easy to be naturally present and aware. Allowing all parts of yourself to work together in harmony can be incredibly empowering. Whether during pregnancy, labor and delivery, or just being a mom, there will be moments when you'll need to draw from a deep reservoir of strength. You can cultivate the depth of this strength both mentally and physically, ideally training both together.

Bridging Physical and Mental Strength

In her TEDx Talk, Amy Morin LCSW said that "If you want to be mentally strong, you need good habits like practicing gratitude." This same advice can be applied to labor and delivery. Choosing to practice gratitude and letting go of old hurts and resentments can help with your mental resilience. Mental resilience is incredibly important for labor and delivery because, as we know from the world of sports psychology, the mind often gives up before the body. Very often when we are training at the gym or going for a power walk, we might tell ourselves *That's enough, I'm done* when in reality our bodies are more than capable of doing another set of lunges or walking an extra quarter mile. Finding gratitude for our strong, healthy bodies can often give us the extra push we need to help the body physically.

Olympic athletes understand the principle of training the mind. Olympic gold medal-winning gymnast Shannon Miller said, "The physical aspect of the sport can only take you so far. The mental aspect has to kick in, especially when you're talking about the best of the best." Although delivery is not a competition, it is very much like a marathon, except that you don't know how long it is going to last or which training skill you will utilize the most. You might need to rely heavily on flexibility, strength, pelvic floor power, meditation, breath work, or most likely on all of the above to one degree or another.

Giving birth is an amazing experience; like for an athletic event, there are months of preparation for the big day. Training your muscles week by week is not just increasing your physical and mental strength and endurance. Each time you make the decision to get up and get moving, whether it's for your yoga practice or for a quick walk with a friend, you are creating good physical habits. Those healthy decisions started with a mental decision: to follow the instinct of health and wellness even though your bed was really comfortable or the couch felt extra inviting that day.

In my classes, I teach that one form of strength can inform another. What I mean by this is that working on your mental strength can help increase your physical strength. A common exercise I do is to have the class hold Warrior

2 just a little bit longer than is comfortable. The reason for this is that the mental endurance you start to build will help you for your baby's birth day. You will already be well versed in the art of endurance. This is a powerful tool to have in your toolbox as you prepare to meet your baby.

Keep in mind that there are times when you also need to have the strength to let go. I have met many moms who have their heart set on a particular type of birth, but things don't always go as planned. If you want to have a vaginal delivery but a C-section is called for, then having the strength to let go of your vision for your baby's birth is a form of emotional strength. Your heart might be set on one outcome, but safety might necessitate another. I believe that your mind, body, and heart can all work in harmony to provide you with the strength you need to make the decisions that are right for you and your baby.

Releasing Fear

Ina May Gaskin, an internationally recognized midwife and expert on maternal care, has written and spoken on the topic of helping moms relax naturally in childbirth. Gaskin teaches women (and men) how to reduce the fear associated with birth. Some of her techniques were inspired by Dr. Grantly Dick-Read, who wrote *Childbirth without Fear*. Dr. Dick-Read, who wrote extensively on the topic of releasing fear of labor and delivery, believed that unbearable labor pain in childbirth was almost always a result of fear. Ina May Gaskin teaches many different ways to help women release fear and anxiety; some of these, as well as tips from doulas and yoga teachers, are included in the following list.

- Natural or soft lighting, because the mother's eyes dilate during birth
- Figure eight movement or hip circles on a stability ball
- Swaying in water
- Dancing
- Humor
- Kissing
- Meditation
- Visualization

Off to the Hospital

Having the right gear for the hospital is important. Be sure to take the following items with you:

- Stability or birthing ball (this can help baby get into the proper position for labor, and can also be used to stretch your lower back)
- Athletic shoes (you might want to take a walk to help induce labor)
- Essential oils (lavender oil encourages calm)
- Robe
- Slippers
- Dry shampoo
- Disposable underwear
- Nursing bra
- Lip balm
- Two outfits for baby to come home in
- Baby blankets (most hospitals will give you extra)

Many of these can help you feel good in your body. Kissing your partner for example, might bring feelings of comfort and connection. Knowing what to expect, how to breathe during labor, and how to push can take away some of the fear and anxiety that are normal, especially for first-time moms. Remember that women have been having babies since the beginning of time, and that your body knows how to have a baby. You can trust your body. But if you and your baby need a little bit of help to get baby from your tummy to your arms, that's OK too.

Choosing Your Birth Path

Have you ever heard someone say *natural birth* when they really meant *vaginal delivery*? I've heard it a lot. To clarify, natural birth means drug free, no epidural and Pitocin. *Vaginal delivery* is self-explanatory, but many of us feel a little shy about using this term. Our Puritan roots in the United States might make us a little uncomfortable using the word *vaginal*, but it is the correct term, and it is important to know that, so that when you are creating your birth plan you are clear on all of the terminology. Vaginal delivery requires pushing. All of the strength you have cultivated in your body, mind, and heart over the last 40 weeks will help you to push.

Vaginal delivery is another instance in which Hollywood has given us a view of birth that is not always accurate. In most movies, you will see a woman lying on her back with her feet in stirrups to deliver her baby. While this is one way of delivering, it is not the only way. In fact, for many centuries, women squatted to allow gravity to help them as they pushed. The 17th-century French king Louis XIV wanted to see the birth of his baby and did not want his view obstructed by the birthing stool that was often used at that time. To accommodate the king, the woman was laid on her back so he could watch his child being born. Little by little, this became a more standard practice that has stayed with us for centuries.

Kneeling, squatting, leaning over something (such as the side of an inflatable tub, in the case of a water birth) are all options for delivering your baby. Many hospitals offer a birthing bar. The bar can be used to hold onto while squatting, or even to put up a foot while in a semireclined position. Epidurals can help significantly with pain management, but it is important to know how the medication affects your body. An epidural reduces the number of positions available to you for giving birth; your legs will be numb, so squatting would no longer be an option.

You might be thinking, *How do I choose what position to give birth in?* While it would be ideal to plan to squat (so gravity can help you), if your baby is posterior (sunny side up), you may have better success delivering on all fours. In other words, you may not know what position is called for until you are pushing. Your doctor and midwife can help you find the best position for delivery, and staying in tune with your body's feedback will help you find what works for you and your baby. As you already know by now, your body's feedback during pregnancy is anything but subtle. You will know right away if you have found the right position.

Once it is time to push, you will call on your pelvic floor strength. Remember all of those Kegels and pelvic floor exercises you've been doing for the better part of a year? Now is the time to put all of that training into action. Your powerful pelvic floor will help to push as you coordinate your breathing with a bearing-down action. You have also been practicing yogic breathing and exhaling on the exertion during exercise. All of these tools and more are available to you during labor and delivery. Breath work, strength, flexibility, and endurance are all at your disposal as you prepare to meet your baby.

You might be asking, *What if I need a C-section?* The fact is that C-sections may either be planned months in advance or be called for at the last minute. Reasons for planning a C-section ahead of time include previous C-section, placenta issues, mom's chronic health condition, breech baby, or multiples. The last-minute C-section is referred to as an emergency C-section. An emergency C-section is performed when there is a complication after labor has already begun. Examples of reasons for needing an emergency C-section include fetal distress, prolonged labor, and umbilical cord prolapse (the cord drops into the vagina ahead of the baby).

C-sections tend to be a polarizing, almost political issue in our country. There are folks who think that the reason for the high rate of C-sections in this country is that doctors prefer a quick, scheduled procedure over a vaginal delivery because it is more convenient for them. On the other hand, there are women who schedule a C-section without it being a medical necessity. There are stories of women who have an elective C-section to accommodate their travel schedules or final exams or because they're afraid of complicated deliveries or long, painful labor. The British tabloids have called such women "too posh to push."

Whatever your stance is on C-section, the reality is that sometimes babies need help getting into this world. If you are having a C-section, whether planned or emergency, you might wonder if all the exercise you did over the last nine months was for naught. The mamas in my classes who have had C-sections have consistently reported that in addition to exercise helping

Placenta Encapsulation

The first time I heard about a woman ingesting her placenta was on a reality show. I thought for sure that the producers had told her to talk about it for shock effect. Now that I have been in the world of birth for many years, I have learned that placenta encapsulation is an ancient technique that is popular in Chinese medicine. If you choose to encapsulate your placenta, someone who specializes in the technique will most likely pick up your placenta right after you have given birth and take it away on dry ice. The placenta is then steamed, dehydrated, ground up, and enclosed in a capsule. There are few studies with hard science on the benefits, but there are many anecdotal reports of benefits, including

- increased release of oxytocin,
- decreased postpartum depression levels,
- increased energy levels, and
- faster restoration of iron levels.

with the pregnancy (such as feeling strong, or less back pain), it also helps them with recovery. A C-section is major abdominal surgery: The abdominal wall is cut to allow baby to come into this world. Not only do the abdominal muscles need to heal but the pelvic floor muscles need to heal too. All of those Kegels are not just for pushing; they also help hold the weight of your baby throughout the pregnancy. The muscles of the perineum still need to recover after holding the weight of a baby for 40 weeks. "The healthier that you are going into surgery, the quicker the recovery," says Rajiv B. Gala, MD, the American College of Obstetricians and Gynecologists' physician-at-large.

Birth Stories

The following birth stories include my own story and the stories of women I have worked with. The exception is Kim's story, a close family member who had her baby over 20 years ago. Her story is of particular interest because she was on the forefront of prenatal exercise; she taught step aerobics through-out her pregnancy. Taking step aerobics, let alone *teaching* step aerobics, while pregnant was very progressive for the 1990s. Fast forward to today, when we have many options for prenatal exercise and much clearer exercise safety guidelines for pregnancy and beyond. You will see that in each story, exercise was an empowering factor for the woman, and that each one of us has a unique and beautiful story. Spoiler alert: Each one has a happy ending.

Desi's Story: Vaginal Delivery With Medical Intervention

In September of 2007, I was 39 weeks pregnant and knew that my baby would come soon. The first Sunday of the month, my husband and I went to spiritual services. We attend services at the Lake Shrine Temple in the Pacific Palisades, which was built by Parmahansa Yogananda. Yogananda was one of the first teachers responsible for bringing yoga to the United States, and the grounds of the Lake Shrine have symbols of all of the world religions. I was so happy to be there and to have the monk bless my very big belly. Later that day, I went for a swim, which was really just my husband dragging me happily around the pool. After the swim, I fell asleep for several hours.

Around 11 P.M., I woke up with a huge gush of water between my legs. It felt like a water balloon had popped. I realized that my water had broken and I called for my husband. He was delighted and nervous and called the doctor. I took a shower while my husband chatted with the doctor, and I could hear his feet pacing. The moment that I got out of the shower he said, "Let's go to the hospital." I laughed and said, "I need to blow my hair out." Yes, I had a moment of vanity and did not want to show up at the hospital looking like a wet poodle.

My husband continued to pace, and much to my amazement I was very calm, as the contractions felt like nothing more than mild menstrual cramps. We drove to the hospital and the doctor on staff wanted to test to see if my amniotic sac had broken, or if I had peed myself in the bed. *What the…?* were the words in my mind; I knew that I had not peed myself. Of course, they soon found out that my water had broken, and I found out that I was not dealing with familiar territory. The staff were all unfamiliar to me, and my husband and I were novices at navigating labor and delivery. Luckily for us, one of my best friends, Lori Bregman, had recently become a doula (she is now a very well-known doula and author), and she arrived at the hospital about an hour later.

By now it was about 3 A.M., and the nurse on duty said that she wanted to give me Pitocin to "get labor going." Apparently I was only dilated at about a 4, and she said, "When your water breaks, you have to give birth within 24 hours." The Pitocin contractions were much more intense and I asked for an epidural. After the epidural, the pain subsided, and I was able to take a little nap. I woke up to beeping because my baby's heartbeat was irregular. I had recently seen the movie *The Business of Being Born*, and was concerned that I was on the medical intervention cycle that leads to a C-section. The nurse on duty said, "Don't worry, honey, we will get you a C-section." The look of terror in my eyes was a signal to my doula to step in. My doula knew that I did not want a C-section unless absolutely necessary, because my baby was in what is called OFP (optimal fetal positioning); his head was down, with his back to my belly, and in a good position for delivery.

Lori asked the nurse on duty when her shift was over. The nurse told Lori that she was on for another five minutes or so, and I will never forget Lori saying "You can leave now." I was so relieved, and I could feel the power shifting back from the nurse to my husband and me. I truly appreciate the amazing and well-intentioned medical community, but this particular nurse at this particular moment was not the right fit. Soon the doctor on staff came in and turned the Pitocin down. My son's heart rate normalized and I took another nap.

Around 3 P.M. I felt the intense need to vomit. Then I thought I needed to run to the ladies room. It was when I said, "You have to let me up, I need to go to the bathroom" that my doula and a new, fantastic nurse looked at each other and said, "Time to push." I did not know that during labor and delivery, it is very common to feel like you need to use the restroom, which makes perfect sense because your body is preparing to bear down and push. As they started to coach me on how to breathe and push, I realized that I could not feel anything from the waist down. As it turns out, the staff had forgotten to further turn down my epidural, and I was completely numb.

At that moment my amazing ob/gyn Dr. Betty Lee arrived and took control of the situation. (By the way, it is amazing how many doctors know exactly when to arrive to "catch" the baby!) She immediately asked the nurse to turn down the epidural, and she reminded me that I am strong. At that moment, all of my years of muscle memory kicked in. I knew that I had the strength to push, and if I could just envision the muscles that I needed to use to push, then I could do it. I turned my attention inward and started to imagine the muscles pushing, and in my mind I was talking to my baby and telling him, *I am ready to meet you, I love you.* Externally I had a lot of help. My husband was behind my upper back and helping me to push from the top down. I specifically asked him to stay "north of the equator," because I was scared that he would faint. I am so glad that I did, because in addition to him helping to support my back, I could feel his reassuring hand behind my heart center. My doula had one foot, and the nurse had the other foot, and they pushed my feet toward me to help me bear down. In the middle and totally ready to catch my baby was my awesome ob. After about 40 minutes of my active pushing, Cruz Roman Bartlett entered the world, and I fell in love at first sight.

JP's Story: Natural, Drug-Free Delivery

My boyfriend and I had an unplanned pregnancy in 2016. My greatest fear at the time was childbirth, so I was not only thrown off by this unexpected pregnancy, but was also terrified of my duty at the end of the pregnancy. I knew I had to do something to overcome my fear. I began to look for anything to help me stay present. My ob/gyn recommended that I sign up for prenatal yoga, and it was the best advice ever.

I felt connected and at peace after enrolling in Desi's prenatal yoga class. I began to learn that even though my pregnancy was unexpected, there were many women who planned their pregnancies and yet shared the same fears that I had. When we would open up and talk during our exercises, the compassion and advice that filled the room always settled my nerves. I continue to advise all of my friends that if they're going to do anything during pregnancy, they must do prenatal yoga. Not only was I building a strong body for birthing, my mind was becoming stronger, more aware, and more centered through our meditations and conversations.

During the last few months of pregnancy, I had complications. My platelet count was low and continued to drop over the last few weeks leading up to my due date, which meant I likely could not have an epidural unless the platelet counts jumped back up. If it weren't for prenatal yoga, my mind would have been a mess, racing and trying to find a sense of control in the situation. Instead, I found a sense of peace and presence in the fact that my baby would help me birth him, and that all would happen the way that it should. The mindfulness and calm that I learned in prenatal yoga class helped me to stay present and pacify my fears.

Additionally, over the last few months of my pregnancy, the doctors began to notice that the baby's abdominal circumference seemed to be proportionally smaller than the rest of his body; they were concerned that my placenta was failing. I was scheduled to be induced a week early; however my platelet counts were still low, which meant I would have two options if things remained the same. I would either have an induced birth with no option of an epidural, or I would have a Cesarean. Both options were not appealing to me, and I struggled with fear. But, I remembered Desi and my classmates, and it was the one thing that helped me the most throughout the remainder of my pregnancy. I was put on bed rest for the last two months of my pregnancy. That didn't make things easier in terms of my racing thoughts, but I was so thankful for the sense of peace and calm that I learned.

The week of my scheduled induction arrived, and I took every bit of advice to try to get labor going myself. My doctor did a membrane sweep in hopes that it would put me into labor sooner. I took walks, ate spicy foods, had sex, had induction massages, and drank the teas. I tried almost everything that might get labor going. I began to talk to my baby and asked him to please come early. A few days before my scheduled induction, my platelet counts spiked back up to a level that would allow me to have an epidural. I couldn't have been happier with the news! As a result, I felt ready and eager for labor, to avoid any invasive procedures.

Two days before my scheduled induction, I was lucky enough to wake up in the middle of the night and go into labor naturally. I labored at my home with my amazing and supportive boyfriend for the first 11 hours of what would be a 22 hour delivery process. When we arrived at the hospital, I was so proud of myself for being 3.5 centimeters dilated and having stayed at home for so long during my labor. I had the most incredible, empowering, and positive birthing experience. I felt like a warrior woman, and I was so excited to meet my baby boy, and not be pregnant anymore. I manifested my wishes for a natural birth into a reality, with my presence, calm, and hard work. I do believe that I went into labor naturally because I helped my body and my baby prepare for the big day. I believe that my mindfulness, readiness, and sense of empowerment were the reasons that I had a positive and natural birthing experience. Any sense of fear was absent during those 22 hours, even though there were a few complications that would have terrified me prior to taking Desi's prenatal yoga classes. I was not only facing my fears about birth, I was doing it fearlessly. I was even shocking myself with my sense of calm, presence, and strength. Not to mention my body was physically strong, and ready for labor. I pushed my son out faster than the medical team expected, and I had to wait for my doctor to arrive. I have Desi's squat intervals to thank for that! I know that without Desi, my mindful ob/gyn, doula, friends from prenatal yoga, the man who is now my loving husband, and family, I would not have had this incredible and empowering birthing experience. I am eternally grateful for all of them.

Natiya's Story: High-Risk Delivery

I was halfway through medical school when I found out we were going to be blessed with our second child. My first pregnancy and birth had gone very smoothly thanks to a consistent yoga practice with Desi Bartlett, so I knew that making time for exercise and breath work were going to be central to my healthy pregnancy plan once again. Still, I wondered if my supermom skills were going to be tested by raising a four-year-old, being pregnant during school, continuing my health and fitness photography business, and prioritizing staying happy and healthy during the pregnancy and birthing process.

Ironically, I was taking a course on prenatal medicine when I got a call from a nurse to discuss the results of my second trimester ultrasound. I had just gotten through the module on delivery complications, so I knew exactly what risks were present when she told me that my baby had a double vessel umbilical cord instead of a triple. This meant that instead of two arteries bringing blood from baby back to the mom, there was one. In most cases, the single artery widens and makes up for the lack of the second and there are no complications. However, because of the possible reduced blood flow, baby can receive less oxygen, and monitoring during pregnancy and delivery is crucial. Babies with double vessel cords can become tired during delivery and risk having trouble moving through the canal, so hospital births are recommended over home births.

My birth plan completely changed when I found out that my baby had a double vessel cord. The yoga and breath work Desi taught me were an even more important part of my daily routine because I wanted to keep baby and me fully oxygenated and toxin free. I was in hard labor for over 30 hours, my baby was at risk of shoulder dystocia, the C-section team had been called in, and suddenly there were over a dozen medical professionals at my bedside. I asked for one more try to birth my baby without surgery and with a big yogi breath and a great deal of faith, my baby girl was born with no complications . . . we named her Grace, and she is amazing!

Demetra's Story: Empowered C-Section

Loukas Alexandros Burkhardt was born on March 7, 2018, 8 pounds 12 ounces, and 22 inches long, and a week and a half past my due date. What I learned throughout this pregnancy and labor and delivery is that although you can plan all you want, things will happen as they are meant to happen and when they are meant to happen. My pregnancy was great. I experienced the typical first trimester exhaustion and morning sickness, but then once I entered the second trimester, they both subsided. I was lucky to be able to continue working out, especially yoga and Pilates, which not only helped me continue to build strength, but also prepared me for labor, delivery, and my recovery.

I had every intention of delivering baby Loukas naturally, but he had a different plan in mind. He was a stubborn little fella, and it began in the womb! After I passed my due date by more than a week, my doctor decided it was time for a bit of assistance and she scheduled me for an induction. I arrived at the hospital a bit nervous, as ready as I could possibly be (but are we ever totally ready?), and excited to finally meet this little man who would forever change my life.

Everything began around 10 A.M. on March 6, and slowly throughout the day, the hospital staff increased the level of Pitocin to intensify my contractions and (hopefully) help the dilation progress. As the contractions strengthened, I found myself really focusing on my breath, thanks to my yoga practice. Breathing through the pain, along with shifting my positions, which I learned in prenatal yoga, really helped take away the edge and keep my mind focused on the end result. At about 8 P.M., I realized it was time for the epidural. I had contemplated whether or not I was going to get one, but I spoke to the midwife and reached a point where I knew it was the right thing to do. As I was hoping that the epidural would relax my muscles a bit more and help the dilation, the night went on. After a few episodes through the night where the baby's heart rate dropped, the hospital staff along with my doctor decided to decrease the amount of Pitocin. Despite what was happening around me, I had my family there for support, and I knew I was in great hands with the staff and felt assured that everything would be OK.

By late morning, I had not dilated any further, and without the Pitocin, my contractions had slowed down. Loukas had other plans. At around 10 A.M. on Tuesday, March 7, my doctor decided it was time to schedule a C-section. Although nervous, I knew at this point that this was the path I had to follow, and honestly, I was OK with it. My priority was the baby and his well-being, and I was surrounded by an exceptional team.

I was scheduled for the C-section at 1 P.M.; however, once again, little Loukas had a different plan in mind. Given the circumstances, the hospital staff decided it was best to speed up the process and go ahead with the C-section. Loukas had spoken to us in his way—this is how he was going to make his entrance into the world. When we got to the operating room, the doctors decided to wait for my doctor while they prepped me. She arrived and I knew everything was going to work out OK. The whole procedure was quick and the team, and of course my significant other who was at my side the whole time, put me at ease. It was a bit strange at first because when the doctor pulled out the baby at 1:09 P.M., I heard him cry but I couldn't see him. Dad got to run over and meet him first and cut the umbilical cord. Meanwhile I was able to listen to everything that was going on as the doctor finished the surgery. And then they brought him over to me.

I can't explain the overwhelming emotions I felt when I finally got to meet Loukas. I was filled with tears of joy, excitement, and a love I had never before felt. He was finally here—healthy, beautiful, and absolutely perfect. I was a mom. We were parents. Our son had arrived!

I spent the next couple of days at the hospital recovering. The surgery had gone extremely well and I was healing relatively quickly. In fact, I was up walking around almost immediately. Even the nurses were impressed. The scar was minimal, thanks to my fantastic doctor. I attribute the speedy recovery to the strength and endurance that I had built up prior to and throughout the pregnancy. By Saturday morning, I was ready to go home with a new addition to my family!

One of the most important things that I learned and that continued to resonate throughout this experience was acceptance. I learned to accept what was happening to me, the physical and emotional changes, the hormones, the ups and downs, and although it was not always easy at times, I learned to embrace it all. After all, I was growing a human! And that's not just remarkable but a miracle and one of the greatest blessings in life. I also learned to accept that the baby will come when he is ready (as he did), and in the manner in which he was destined. In my case, it was a Cesarean section, and that's OK. Loukas is here. He's happy, he's healthy, and he's the greatest gift of all—and that's all that matters. I couldn't ask for anything more.

Shawna's Story: Natural, Drug-Free Vaginal Delivery in Water at a Birthing Center

As soon as I found out I was pregnant, I knew intuitively that I wanted to have a water birth. As a practitioner of yoga and feminine movement with a holistic outlook on life, I felt this was the natural decision for me. As an emergency room nurse, my husband was initially skeptical but came on board once we met our midwife, who also used to be a labor and delivery nurse. After discussing it, we decided that we wanted to give birth at the birthing center rather than at home.

At exactly 38 weeks, I began to have contractions at five o'clock in the morning. They were inconsistent and I assumed it was false labor, but I let my midwife and doula know just in case. By late morning, the contractions still varied in timing but had started to intensify in sensation, and I knew it was the real thing. Using my exercise ball and the breathing exercises I had learned in birth class, I labored at home until late afternoon. The contractions started to get stronger and come closer together, and I told my husband that we needed to book it to the birthing center. Once we got there, my midwife checked me and I was already 7 to 8 centimeters dilated.

My doula arrived, and together with my husband massaged me, held my hands, and breathed with me as I moved from the birthing tub to the bathroom when I got too warm, and then to the bed. I had made a playlist while I was pregnant, and music was softly playing in the background. I felt primal, each contraction bringing about low, guttural moans. The contractions passed through me like powerful waves. As the sun started to set, I began to feel the urge to push, but my water had not yet broken. My midwife suggested that I sit on the toilet to allow gravity to do its work, and as soon as I moved from the bed my water broke during a contraction so powerful it brought me to my knees. I got back into the tub, now fully dilated, and within 30 minutes of my pushing—the most intense sensations I had ever experienced—my husband caught our baby boy in the water.

We were immediately in awe of this tiny, perfect little human being. My husband and I enjoyed about two hours of uninterrupted skin to skin bonding with Tyson, and watched in amazement as he wriggled his way to my breast to feed for the first time. After he was weighed, checked, and bundled up, our new little family headed home just four and a half hours after I gave birth. Pretty crazy! I was so lucky to have the birth that I envisioned. And now that I have joined the motherhood tribe, I have also gained an inherent respect for all the strong, powerful women who have given birth.

Kim's Story: The Coolest Natural, Drug-Free Vaginal Delivery

At the 40-hour mark, the ob/gyn came into my room and said we'd likely have to take the baby by C-section. I asked if the baby was in distress and he said, "Well, no, not yet but you're still only at two centimeters." I told him that I had not endured 40 hours of labor to let him take the baby by C-section now.

I had continued my workouts and taught aerobics throughout my pregnancy so I was confident in my ability to have the natural, drug-free birth that I had envisioned. For the better part of two days, I had been breathing deeply and finding strength by going to my center and quieting myself, but I was tiring. I could hear another woman screaming and all I could think was that I just didn't want to waste my energy that way. My husband had returned home to rest for a bit and I felt quite alone.

After the frustrated ob/gyn left, a nurse came into my darkened and quiet room wearing an old-fashioned nurse's cap and a crisp white uniform. She asked if I was willing to try something different and I said, "Absolutely!" She disconnected the monitors and had me get out of the bed and straddle a hard-backed wooden chair. My only job was to relax everything I could and expand my belly as much as possible. Meanwhile, she took the heel of her hand and firmly pressed it into my lower back, pushing up toward my shoulder blades repeatedly. It was not comfortable and I was challenged to try and relax against the strong pressure. She gently explained to me that my baby was lying transverse and that we wanted to make her a bit uncomfortable so that her head would find the birth canal. I didn't know the sex of my baby yet but didn't think anything of the nurse's use of the feminine pronoun at the time. I really don't know how much time passed but at some point I felt an intense pulling and pressure and the nurse said, "There she goes. It won't be long now." And with that she helped me back into bed and left.

I went from 2 to 10 centimeters so quickly that the nurse who checked me gasped. They had to call the ob/gyn back from dinner at an outside restaurant, and he barely made it before she was crowning. "Don't push!" he kept yelling at me. The incredible relief and overwhelming awesomeness of seeing my daughter's arrival was the most rewarding feeling I'd ever experienced. I asked later where that helpful nurse was who got me out of bed and on that wooden chair to work her magic. I very much wanted to thank her. But the ob/gyn and the nurses had no idea know who I was talking about. They told me that they'd had an emergency in another room that had taken several hours of their time but they hadn't seen anyone around my birthing suite. I was informed that if the monitors had been disconnected the alarms would have gone off at the nurse's station and that there wasn't a single wooden chair on the entire floor. I told them what she looked like and mentioned her uniform. They rolled their eyes, and one laughed out loud and said "Oh, sweetie, nurses haven't worn uniforms like that in years!"

Note: This story was shared with me by a close family member. In speaking with her, I concluded that it is quite possible that she was in a very deep meditative state. She believes that the nurse who helped her was from the angelic realm. While this sounds kind of out there, many believe that birth is a time when the veil between the physical world and the divine is lifted. Whatever your personal beliefs are, this is a cool story that illustrates the ability to go deep within your own consciousness during birth and find the tools to empower you.

Mommy Move

Hip Sways in the Shower

When you feel the onset of labor, whether it is the beginning of consistent contractions or if your water has broken, you will most likely still have a bit of time at home before you head to the hospital or the birthing center. You can use this time to prepare your body for the amazing experience of labor and delivery with simple hip sways in the shower. If you are delivering your baby at home, you will have more time available to enjoy this movement for as long as it feels good.

Stand in a warm shower with your face pointed toward the wall with the showerhead. Place your hands at the level of your hips and walk your feet back slightly until you can hinge at your hips. You will recognize this shape as Puppy Pose from chapter 5. Have your feet hip width apart and allow your hips to sway from side to side slowly as the stream from the shower flows down your spine like a waterfall. The warm water will help to relax you and will feel like a gentle massage on your back. The gentle swaying from side to side will help baby to move into the birth canal. Close your eyes and envision your baby in OFP. You can also tell your baby that you are celebrating his or her arrival. Note: This is not intended to be a workout. This is a gentle invitation for your baby to start to move down in preparation for birth as well as an opportunity to soothe your nervous system.

Information No One Tells You

Curbing Nausea

No one told me that when your baby is about to be born, it is very common to feel the need to expel. This can be either the urge to vomit or the sensation of needing to use the restroom. Vomiting can sometimes be a reaction to an epidural, or it can simply be a sign that you are transitioning into active labor. Either way, we can all agree that vomiting is no fun. Here are some simple steps that you can take to help quell queasiness.

- Stay hydrated; you can chew on ice chips, drink water, or eat a popsicle.
- Eat very light, bland foods.
- Put a few drops of ginger tincture in your water.
- If you are at home, have your partner or midwife diffuse peppermint essential oil.

Love-Your-Baby Visualization

Holding Your Baby

Close your eyes and envision your beautiful baby in optimal positioning, with the head down and spine to your belly. Start an internal conversation with your baby. Share with your baby all of your excitement to meet him or her (or both if you have opposite-sex twins). Let your little one know that when he or she is ready to enter the world, you are ready too, and that you have been waiting to cradle your baby in your arms. Feel the love from your heart center traveling through the channels of your arms, and place your hands on your abdomen. Try to sense, see, and feel your love emanating from your hands to your baby. Breathe deeply and stay receptive to the feedback of your baby and your body. Notice if there has been a subtle or dramatic shift, and know that as you gently return your consciousness to the present moment, you will soon meet your baby.

Fun Foods

Contributed by Victoria Dodge, creator of Nourishment Now

This smoothie is loaded with nourishing nutrients like healthy fats from the coconut oil and almond butter, potassium and fiber from the banana and dates, and vitamin C and iron from the spinach, not to mention vitamin E from the almond milk. Feel free to add a scoop of your favorite plant-based protein powder to give it an extra boost of protein.

Labor and Delivery Nourishing Smoothie

>   1 cup almond milk
>
>   1 frozen banana
>
>   2 tablespoons almond butter
>
>   2 or 3 dates
>
>   1 teaspoon coconut oil
>
>   Handful of spinach
>
>   1/4 to 1/2 cup water for desired consistency

Combine ingredients in blender. Blend until smooth. Refrigerate the remainder.
Yield: *2 servings*

Practices for Recovery and Results

New Mama Recovery Workout

Congratulations, mama! I know that your body, mind, and heart have been forever changed by the amazing experience of pregnancy, labor, delivery, and birth. Everyone has a unique experience, and the same woman can have different experiences with each pregnancy.

The body's recovery is very important before you start to engage in exercise beyond the demands of daily life, such as lifting your baby, walking, or laundering baby clothes. As you honor this time of transitioning into the role of mother, there are specific, gentle moves and practices that can help promote a sense of well-being as you recover your strength. The focus of this chapter is on helping to promote healing while you bond with your beautiful baby.

Your Body During Recovery

If your baby was delivered vaginally, the typical recovery time is around four weeks. At the four-week mark, you will go to see your ob/gyn or midwife and make sure that your body is healing. For C-section, a six-week recovery time is more the norm, as it is major abdominal surgery and the body needs extra time to heal. Your health care practitioner is responsible for checking to see that everything is healing properly.

It is natural for there to be some tearing if you had a vaginal delivery, and these delicate tissues need some time to heal. This is also the time that you are starting to get the hang of breastfeeding (if that is your path; no judgment either way, breast or bottle), and your breasts might feel heavy or sore. Your abdominal area is also healing; some changes have happened here to make space for your baby. Let's take a look at some of these powerful changes, starting with your belly, the place that was your baby's home.

Abdomen

Your belly has been your baby's home for about the last 40 weeks. If your baby was born via C-section, there is the issue of wound care and making sure that the incision has healed properly. There are different types of

C-sections these days, including traditional and gentle, and your physician may have used an O C-section retractor. Each woman's experience is a little bit different, and healing rates vary.

Another issue you may experience postpartum is diastasis recti (DR), a common condition involving a separation of the two sides of the abdominal muscles. Normally these muscles are connected by strong collagen connective tissue. Describing DR as a separation is a bit misleading; there is always a certain amount of separation because the two sides are connected in the middle underneath the linea alba, that white line that runs from your umbilicus (belly button) down and that often turns black during pregnancy from the shift in hormones. A better way to describe the condition is to say that the quality of this connective tissue can be compromised during pregnancy.

Not always, but very often, I see women who have DR fall into three clear and distinct groups.

▌ The first group is the ultrafit moms who had abs of steel or who teach Pilates. The abs are so tight and so taut that the pressure of the baby growing forward causes a greater separation of the abs. Think of a really tight rubber band being pulled even tighter; eventually something has to give.

▌ The second group is mamas who are deconditioned and are carrying a higher percentage of body fat than is desirable for their health. With these women, there can be excess abdominal fat and a lack of muscle tone before the pregnancy. The muscles are pressed forward by the growth of the baby, and the already lax muscles can get even looser.

▌ The third group in which I often see DR is moms of multiples. Imagine two or three babies growing in the expanding uterus, which then presses forward against the abdominal wall.

It is important to note that there will be a little bit of a separation of the abdominal muscles during the first few hours and days after labor and delivery as your uterus goes through a process called involution. During involution, the uterus is contracting back down from the expanded size to a size that is closer to the size of your fist. So, wait a few weeks before you check to see if you have DR. If you would like to check for DR at home, here are some simple guidelines from my friend and physical therapist Jennifer Wells McCauley, PT, DPT, OCS, PMA-CPT.

1. Begin by lying on your back with your knees bent and feet flat.
2. Place the fingers of one hand, palm facing toward you, at the level of the umbilicus.
3. Slowly lift your head, neck, and shoulders off the floor into a mini crunch position while gently pressing your fingertips down.
4. Assess for gapping or separation between the two rectus halves. It is normal to have from no gap at all up to a one-and-a-half-finger gap

between the two rectus halves. A gap of more than two fingers wide indicates the presence of diastasis recti.

5. Repeat this process at both three fingers above and three fingers below the umbilicus.

It is important to remember that a DR is common in the postpartum period because of the physiological and hormonal changes that occur with pregnancy. It is important to know when to make modifications and when it's best to consult a physical therapist or a medical professional. A gap of less than one and a half fingers is considered normal, and you can proceed with normal abdominal strengthening. A gap of two to three fingers will require modifications with abdominal exercises, and special attention from a certified and experienced yoga instructor or other fitness professional. If you have a gap of more than three fingers, you should see a physical therapist or medical professional; you may require further bracing, taping, or one-on-one instruction to help you with closing the diastasis. In extreme cases, surgery may be warranted, but most DR will recover naturally or with physical therapy.

Pelvic Floor

In addition to making sure that your abdomen is healing, it is important to make sure that the pelvic floor muscles are healing. Very often in the first postnatal checkup, your doctor is checking to see if there are any major issues, such as prolapse. Jennifer Wells McCauley suggests the following as some of the factors to consider in postpartum pelvic floor health.

▪ The type of delivery.
▪ Muscles, ligaments, and tissues may be traumatized.
▪ Partial denervation from compression, stretching, and tearing.
▪ Confused proprioception from Valsalva and from bearing down during childbirth.
▪ Forceps, episiotomy, or inadequate stitching issues.

All of the above can and should be discussed with your doctor, who may not be routinely checking for the tone or the strength of the pelvic floor muscles. Many women know right away if their pelvic floor muscles are weak because any downward pressure can cause bladder leakage. For example, if you feel like you have to pee when you sneeze or when you lift your baby, then speaking with a physical therapist who specializes in treating pelvic floor conditions can be of great help.

If you would like to start recovering the strength and tone of these muscles, try to feel a gentle lift in the pelvic floor during the exercises in the Wake Me Up practice later in this chapter. As you inhale in each exercise, the pelvic floor moves gently down and the abdominal muscles expand. As you exhale, feel the deeper belly muscles draw in and the pelvic floor lift. I like to

Buying the Right Gear

It's important to buy the right gear for postnatal exercise. Here are few items to add to your shopping list.

- A supportive bra that has two separate cups for your breasts to prevent compression of the milk ducts.
- A foam roller to roll out any tension in the connective tissue in your back body and outer thighs.
- Light bladder leakage pads in case you find that you are leaking urine when you exercise, sneeze, or laugh.
- Workout leggings that are high-waisted and offer light compression to help remind your abs to engage.
- Belly bands are optional. If you choose to use a belly band, make sure to protect a C-section incision.

cue a Kegel or an elevator exercise during the exhalation. For example, "As you find the isometric contraction (this is a fancy way of saying contracting without outside movement) of the abdomen, remember to feel the slow and steady lift of the pelvic floor muscles, like an elevator moving from one floor to the next." A good way to remember when to lift the pelvic floor muscles is called the *XX rule* (a mnemonic that kinesiology and biomechanics students use to remember to cue *eXhale on the eXertion*). In this example, you exert the strength of the pelvic floor muscles on the exhalation.

Meditation and Intention for the Recovery Period

It is important to remember that it is not just your body that had the experience of labor and delivery; it was your entire being, including your mind and your heart. I have heard some amazing and inspirational birth stories from the thousands of women I've worked with. But some experiences left the parents feeling disempowered. Take a moment to tap back into the tool of meditation and check in with your innermost self.

Choose a comfortable seated position like Easy Pose and use back support in the form of a wall or your couch. Close your eyes and slow your breath. Begin to scan your body from head to toe. The yogis call this *svadhyaya*, or self-study. Do parts of your body feel tired or need some extra TLC? Are some parts still healing and need rest? Are you already feeling really good and as though life has begun to establish a new rhythm? Try not to judge what comes up: There is no right or wrong, there is only the truth of your experience.

Now easily allow yourself to recall the birth of your beautiful baby. Review the where, when, and who (was in the room). Now, reconnect to the how.

How did your baby enter the world? Did you feel empowered and supported in your choices? Did your doctor or midwife listen to your feedback? Were there moments that scared you? Were there moments that inspired and uplifted you? Again, there is no judgment, especially of yourself.

Lastly, imagine that you can send your love back in time to the you that is experiencing labor and delivery. Look back at this part of yourself with the compassion of a mother's heart. Let your inner gaze be gentle, patient, and understanding of any choices or events that you wish you could rewrite, and try to allow these experiences to inform how you might wish to make changes for future pregnancies (such as being more vocal, asking for pain management or not, having or not having family in the room). If you felt empowered and great, take a moment to connect to those feelings. Again, there is no judgment, just a little self-study and time to process this dramatic life event, the moments that led to you meeting one of the loves of your life, your son or daughter. Slowly let your consciousness come back into the present moment, flutter your eyes open, and if you would like to journal about your experience, take time to do that now. This can be a powerful tool for remembering all the great experiences like holding your baby for the first time, as well as the opportunity to begin to heal experiences that were scary or left you feeling disempowered. Breathe deeply and be truthful with yourself about your feelings. When we know where we are starting from, then we can effectively move in the direction of our intention.

Intention is a buzzword in the mind–body community right now. It sounds really cool and sort of spiritual, but what does it really mean? Intention can be thought of as a determination to act in a certain way, or as our resolve. At the beginning of your yoga practice, it is important to take a moment to set a clear intention. Intentions can be as general as stating the reason you are practicing yoga that day. For example, you might think, *I am inviting flexibility and strength into my body and mind*, or more specifically, *Today as I move through a gentle practice, my intention is to slowly reawaken my core strength without disturbing the site of my C-section incision*. I know that when you are a new mom, there are nights when you might not have had eight hours of sleep, or let's be honest, maybe you had four hours of sleep, nursed your baby, and then had a 20-minute nap before your husband's alarm clock went off. So, if your mind is a little foggy and nothing comes to mind when setting a clear intention, here is a list of intentions that you can choose from:

▌ Calling in strength

▌ Re-energizing my body

▌ Awakening my core muscles

▌ Breathing deeply into motherhood

▌ Breathing deeply into the new rhythm of life

Taking Care of You

Every few years there is a new buzzword or phrase in the mind–body field. Fads come and go, but some broader ideas like mindfulness and clean eating stand the test of time because they contain the wisdom of taking care of ourselves. As a society, we have finally taken the time to recognize that self-care is in and of itself a category that deserves our attention. Self-care can be described as any activity that we do deliberately in order to take care of our mental, emotional, and physical health.

It's clear from this definition that there are as many possibilities for activities to fit into this description as there are moms. Take the time to identify which activities help you to take care of you. When we become moms, everything changes; our bodies, our minds, our hearts, our priorities, and our schedules can all change dramatically as soon as baby is born. It is very important not to put yourself last on the list. When mom takes care of herself, everyone in the family benefits. It's like the old story about not being able to give from an empty cup. It is incredibly important to find something that you can enjoy just for you. Here are some ideas to inspire your own list.

- Meditation and visualization
- A long walk with your best friend
- Date night with your spouse
- Anything that makes you laugh
- Choosing healthy foods that give you energy
- Yoga

Take some time just for you each day. It might be five minutes in the shower with your favorite music playing, or lighting a candle next to your yoga mat to transform your practice into a retreat-style yoga practice. Think of the little things that bring you energy. As a new mother, recovering your strength and taking care of yourself can empower you in this new chapter of life.

Exercise During the Recovery Period

You've received your doctor's clearance to exercise; scanned your body, mind, and heart to see what needs your attention; and set a clear intention. Now it's time to get moving. But what is safe? How do you know if you're doing too much? Just as the body's feedback during pregnancy is anything but subtle, the body also speaks loud and clear when you are a new mom. Listen to your body; if it's screaming for sleep, it is important to honor that. On those days when you feel your energy returning, that's your opportunity to get back into the groove of exercise.

Walking

As during pregnancy, walking is a great way to get moving after you have delivered your beautiful baby. Walking is one of the basic movements that the human body can perform. A great way to begin your reentry into movement is a simple walking schedule that includes an A.M. walk, and a P.M. walk. Bodybuilders and performance athletes call this type of workout *two-a-days*. The CDC recommends that for substantial health benefits, adults should do at least 150 minutes (2 hours and 30 minutes) a week of moderate-intensity aerobic activity, or 75 minutes (1 hour and 15 minutes) a week of vigorous-intensity aerobic activity, or an equivalent combination of moderate- and vigorous-intensity aerobic activity. Aerobic activity should be performed in episodes of at least 10 minutes, and preferably, it should be spread throughout the week.

I know you're probably thinking, *Wait, you want me to start a gentle reentry into exercise with two full workouts a day?!* The workouts I'm encouraging you to do are very brief: a 15-minute walk in the morning with your baby and a 15-minute walk in the evening with your baby, at least five days a week. You can actually walk off a lot of the baby-weight by wearing your baby! And yes, I am aware that *baby-wearing* sounds so LA! The truth is that wearing your baby is an ancient practice shared by women across the globe. In underdeveloped nations, some women need to get back to working the fields or farm very soon after having a baby, so wearing the baby is a necessity for the health and safety of the infant. In other nations, this practice has become a fashion statement with all kinds of beautiful fabrics and patterns available. Finding the right way to secure your baby close to your body is very personal; some women swear by the same carrier that others detest. Here are some important tips to help you choose a baby carrier.

- Make sure that you have the proper fit for your body and for baby.
- Keep baby secure. If you have chosen a wrap-style carrier, lean forward slightly (while supporting baby) and make sure that baby does not fall forward.
- Make sure that baby's head is supported by the carrier. This is especially important for infants.
- If you feel lower back pain or strain, try a different carrier.
- Make sure that you can see your baby's beautiful face. Baby should be able to breathe freely and easily in the carrier.

Remember that there is an adaptation response to training. This means that if we keep working with the same weight all of the time, we plateau in our results. There needs to be a gradual increase in the resistance or weight we are training with, in order to see results. Mother Nature has provided the sweetest, cutest, most precious form of weight there is, in the form of your beautiful baby. Each week as he or she gains a few ounces, you are naturally increasing your strength from the weight of your baby in addition to increasing your cardiovascular endurance from your walking. It is a winning trifecta for mama as she walks off the excess weight, increases strength by wearing baby, and gets to bond with and cuddle baby close to her heart throughout the workout.

Yoga

Yoga is a fantastic tool for recovering your strength, flexibility, balance, good posture, and overall sense of well-being. You have been cleared for exercise, but you are probably a little bit fatigued, and if you are nursing, I don't have to tell you that that is a full-time job. Yoga can be gently introduced into your routine at about six weeks postpartum, or whenever you have clearance from your ob/gyn to exercise. This chapter ends with two recovery workouts that you can enjoy any time of day. These two practices allow you to gently reclaim and rebuild your strength.

Yoga Poses for Abdominal Recovery

After your baby is born, it is important to take the time to rebuild your strength in a gentle and mindful way. The exercises included in this recovery section are inspired by the world of physical therapy. Therapeutic exercises that are often used to help promote DR rehabilitation can also help you reconnect to the feeling of engaging your core. Remember that core strength involves lower back strength, too, and working with these types of exercises will set you up for success, because you will have a baseline of strength before you return to your regular workouts in the coming weeks and months. These exercises can also help you develop functional strength for engaging your core when you are carrying your baby.

Isometric Abdominal Contraction

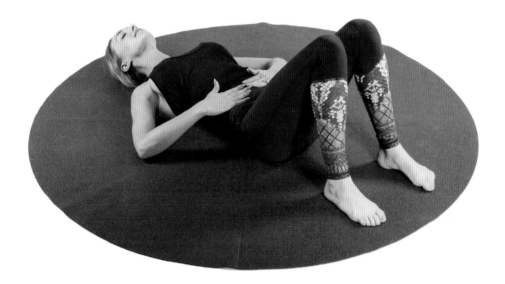

Benefits

This movement awakens the deep abdominal muscles and promotes harmony of the inner cylinder, which includes the diaphragm, the TVA, the pelvic floor, and the lower back.

Feeling

Breathe the feeling of awakening into your lower abdomen. Feel these muscles, which have been working to hold the weight of your baby and your growing body, start to wake up and draw in toward the spine. You are reclaiming this space and reawakening the contractile force with each exhalation.

Instruction

- Begin lying down flat on your back with your feet hip width apart and all ten toes pointed straight forward (make sure not to point the toes in or out).
- Place your hands on your lower abdomen so that you can feel the contraction of the deeper belly muscles (see figure).
- Contract your abdominal muscles by drawing your abdomen in toward the spine and sustain that contraction for 20 seconds.
- It is important to try to feel that the spine is neutral, with no tucking of the pelvis and no pronounced sway in the back. The work is focused and very deep. Make sure not to hold your breath.

Adjustments

If your lower back is tender, it's OK to place a folded blanket beneath your sacrum (that big bone just below the waistband of your pants in back). Make sure that the blanket is neatly folded so as not to create any inconsistencies with the level of support.

Bent-Knee Fallout

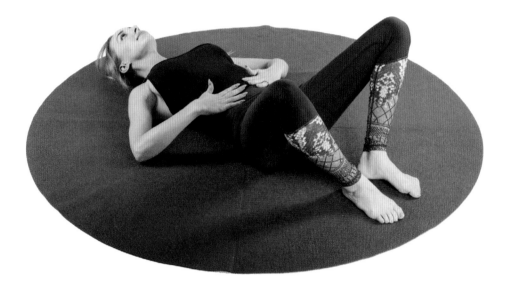

Benefits

This movement provides deep abdominal work as well as helping you learn to coordinate the strength and balance in the pelvic girdle.

Feeling

Envision the hip bones as a set of scales, like in the old-fashioned paintings of the scales of justice. Let the scales be completely even so that they work in harmony and balance, and neither side (especially the stronger side) takes over. Balance is the key to this exercise.

Instruction

▮ Begin by lying flat on your back with your feet hip width apart and all ten toes pointed straight forward (make sure not to point toes in or out).
▮ Place your hands on your lower hip bones (see figure).
▮ Alternately lower one knee out to the side, to a 45 degree angle if possible.
▮ Bring the knee up slowly, and then change sides.
▮ Make sure that the pelvis is not tipping from side to side. Your left hip bone should stay in the same place while the right knee gently falls out to the right. It will take a lot of control to maintain the hip bones in a level position.

Adjustments

As with all floor work, it's OK to have a thin blanket folded underneath your sacrum for padding. This can feel especially good if you have a bony sacrum. Even if you are not super lean, these bones can be prominent and press into the floor. Make the exercise comfortable so you can stick with it and set yourself up for success.

Bridge Pose

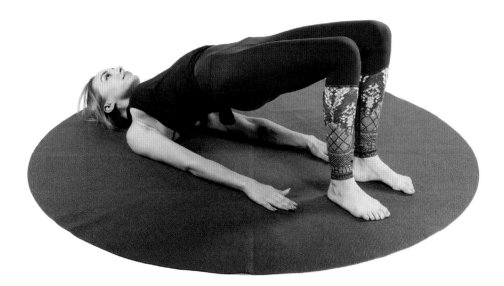

Benefits

This movement strengthens the back of the body through closed chain gluteal stabilization. *Closed chain exercise* refers to movements in which the farthest part of the extremity is in a fixed position. That is a very fancy way of saying that your feet (or your hands in the case of a push-up) do not move while you are performing an exercise. Closed chain exercises are widely used by physical therapists because they are said to be more functional.

Feeling

Bridge Pose can be visualized as crossing a bridge. In this case, you have recently crossed the bridge from pregnancy into motherhood. Feel the shape of the bridge in your body and consider the new bridges that you might be crossing as a mother.

Instruction

- Begin by lying on your back with your feet hip width apart and all ten toes pointing straight forward (make sure not to point toes in or out).
- Bend your knees and softly rest your hands on the floor.
- Lift your hips, feeling your glutes activate, and making sure not to let your knees either bow out or collapse in (see figure).
- Repeat the exercise for 10 repetitions to help build strength in your glutes.

Adjustments

Place a block between your inner thighs so you have something to squeeze. This squeezing in toward the midline will help activate the stabilizers of the thighs and assist with the alignment of the pose.

Unilateral Isometric Hip Flexion

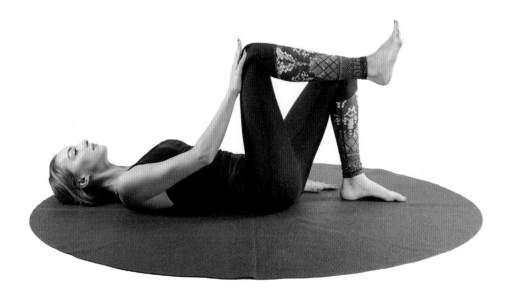

Benefits

This movement strengthens the abdominal muscles.

Feeling

Invite the feeling of balance. It is natural to have one side that is stronger than the other. This is true of the abdominal muscles too. Notice which side is a little bit stronger, and try to bring even more attention and focus to the other side when doing the exercise. Unilateral (one-sided) exercises allow us great insight into the habits of the right and left sides of our bodies. Take the time to invite a greater sense of balance from right to left.

Instruction

- Begin by lying on your back with your feet hip width apart and all ten toes pointing straight forward (make sure not to point toes in or out).
- Place your right hand on top of the right thigh.
- Engage your abs as you lift the right thigh toward you. Firmly press your hand into the top of the thigh, keeping your abs engaged. Try to keep the hips side by side and even (see figure).
- Repeat up to 10 times, and then change sides.

Adjustments

A neatly folded blanket under your lower back can give you some cushion if your lower back feels as though it is pressing into the floor.

Arm-Only Pointer Dog Pose

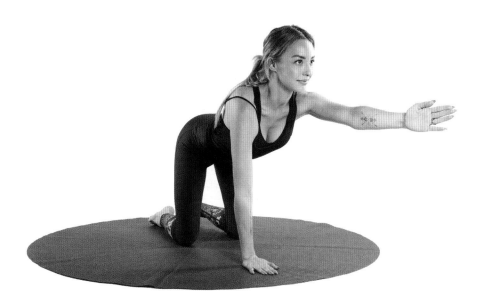

Benefits

This pose awakens core strength and is also beneficial for balance training.

Feeling

Imagine a long line of energy extending forward, like a compass arrow finding true north.

Instruction

- Begin on all fours with hands shoulder width apart and knees hip width apart.
- Inhale and lift the left arm with the thumb pointed to the sky. Find length in the spine as you reach the front hand forward (see figure).
- Make sure that the hips stay level, and feel a lift in the abdomen so that your abs are engaged.
- Keep your neck long with the gaze straight ahead of the yoga mat.
- Enjoy three to five deep breaths, and then change sides.

Adjustments

A folded blanket under the knees can provide cushion. If you have wrist pain or carpal tunnel syndrome, you can practice this pose with your bottom hand in a fist instead of a flat palm.

Prone Bent-Knee Lift

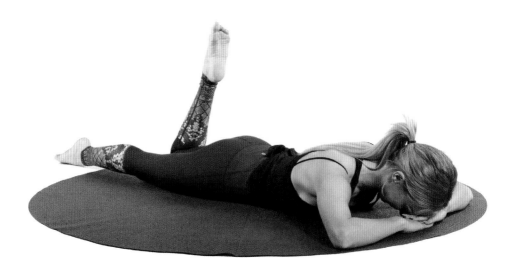

Benefits

This movement creates strength in the lower back, glutes, and hamstrings.

Feeling

Breathe into the strength of the back body and connect to its power. We spend so much time training the muscles we can see in the mirror that sometimes we forget that the powerful back body provides support and structure. Remember to feel the breath in the back of your body. Feel the back ribs expand gently with each inhalation and affirm that even the parts of you that you cannot see are getting stronger.

Instruction

- Lie facedown on your belly with your hands gently folded underneath your forehead to create a soft pillow.
- With your right leg straight on the mat, bend your left knee and slowly lift the left hip. Make sure not to arch the lower back (see figure).
- Alternate sides and work up to 10 to 12 repetitions per side.

Adjustments

A folded blanket underneath your pubic bone provides cushion. It can be helpful to have someone take a picture of you in this exercise, or you can set your smartphone camera on a timer so that you can get visual feedback about your strength and to ensure proper form. You will notice if one hip lifts higher than the other during the lifting part of the exercise or if you are overarching your back. Eventually you will gain the awareness to feel this from the inside out.

Heel Squeeze

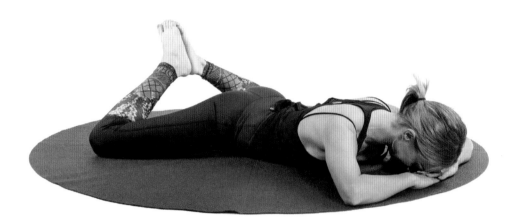

Benefits

This movement helps to train the thighs and glutes and to stabilize the pelvis. It can also help improve pelvic floor strength.

Feeling

Try to feel your lower body strength reawakening after the 40 weeks of pregnancy. For the duration of the pregnancy, lying prone (on your abdomen) is not advised. Now that your baby has been born, enjoy the feeling of lying on the earth and feeling its support as you rebuild your own foundation and base of support.

Instruction

- Lie facedown with your arms folded underneath your forehead to create a pillow.
- Slide your legs out to the side so that your knees are almost straddling your yoga mat.
- Bend your knees and squeeze your heels together (see figure).
- Try to hold the heel squeeze for 10 seconds.
- Repeat the exercise 10 times.

Adjustments

A blanket under the pelvis or knees can provide cushion if you need it.

Straight-Leg Raise

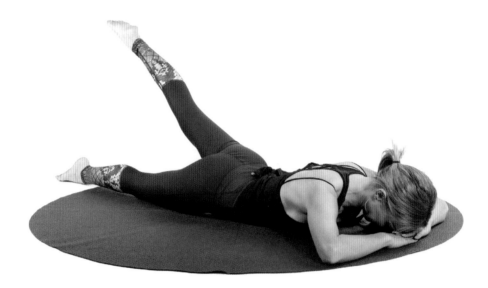

Benefits

This exercise trains the glutes and the hamstrings and helps stabilize the pelvis.

Feeling

Breathe a feeling of strength into your lower body as you lift the legs. Awaken the back of the body with each repetition and feel how these muscles help support your posture as well as supporting your ability to lift your baby.

Instruction

▌ Lie facedown with your arms folded underneath your forehead to create a pillow.
▌ Keep both of your legs straight and avoid overarching your lower back.
▌ Keep the legs as straight as possible as you lift the left leg at the hip (see figure).
▌ Repeat 10 times, and then change sides.

Adjustments

A blanket under the pelvis or knees can provide cushion if you need it.

Forearm Plank Pose

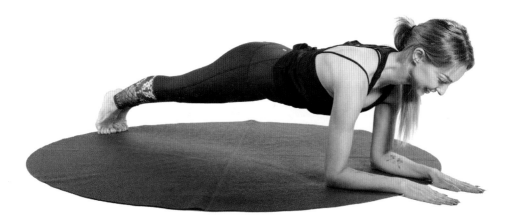

Benefits

This pose cultivates strength in the core muscles including the abs, the lower back, the obliques, and the TVA.

Feeling

Breathe the feeling of strength into your abdomen. Remember that this was your baby's home for 40 weeks. Your baby now has a new home and no longer needs the space in your belly. Thank your belly for creating this space for your little one, and let your body know that it can now begin to draw everything back into the midline, like a corset. This corseting action will help you with your posture.

Instruction

- Begin in Plank Pose but on your forearms with your toes tucked under and your core muscles engaged (see figure).
- Make sure that your hips are not sinking.
- Try to work up to 20 seconds per set, and work up to three sets.

Adjustments

If you are exercising next to your baby, you can set up baby with a blanket at the front of your mat. Look into your baby's eyes and smile. To challenge yourself in this exercise, roll forward and back gently on the toes so that your entire body shifts slightly forward and back. Try to do this while gazing at your baby and see if you can get baby to smile. The added incentive of working for the baby's smile can help bring joy into this intense exercise.

Down Dog Pose
Into Stacked Hip Variation

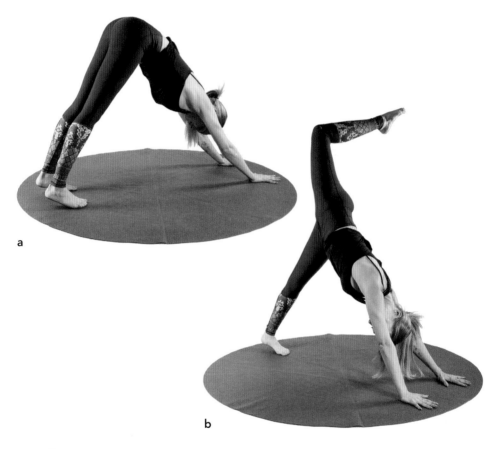

a

b

Benefits

This pose strengthens the upper body and stretches the psoas of the lifted leg.

Feeling

Supporting yourself with three points of contact with the earth in Down Dog chal-lenges your balance and forces your upper body to work harder. This is a great place to start to get comfortable with inversions. An inversion is any pose in which your head is below your heart. Focus on the power and strength of your upper body as you explore this gentle inversion.

Instruction

- Begin on your hands and knees with knees hips width apart.
- Lift your hips and work toward straightening your legs into Down Dog (see figure a).
- Lift the right leg and bend the knee as you work toward stacking the hips, which means keeping them in line with the heels (see figure b).
- Change sides.

Half Sun Salutation With Backbend

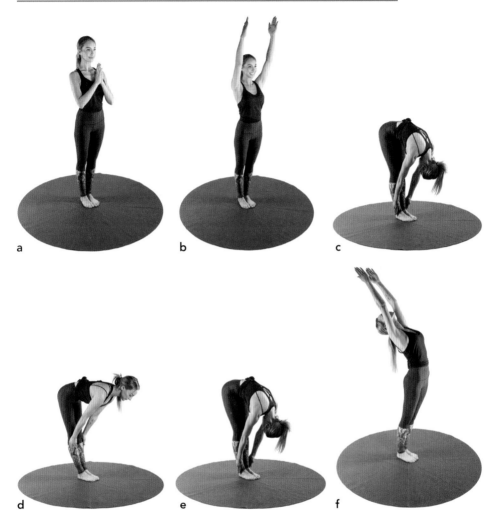

Benefits
This sequence gently warms up the body, especially the core and shoulders.

Feeling
The sequence gives you a sense of inviting warmth and radiance into your body.

Instruction
- Begin standing with your hands in namaste and your feet together (see figure a).
- Inhale with your arms overhead, exhale (see figure b), and take an easy Forward Fold (see figure c).
- Lengthen the spine and rise halfway up (see figure d), then soften into Forward Fold again (see figure e).
- Rise back to standing with a gentle back bend in the thoracic spine (upper body) on the inhale (see figure f).
- Exhale and bring your hands to your heart in namaste (see figure a).

Supported Backbend on Stability Ball

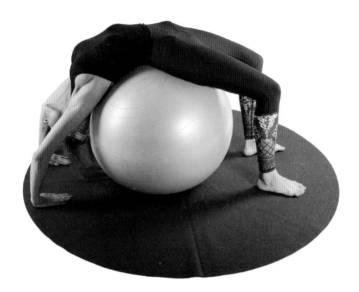

Benefits

This exercise stretches the entire front of the body, including the chest, shoulders, abdomen, and front of the legs.

Feeling

The gift of motherhood often feels as though it opens your heart wide. Take time in this stretch to breathe strength into your heart space and enjoy the feeling of your arms being wide open to receive the gift of this enormous amount of love that has come into your life.

Instruction

❚ Begin seated on top of the stability ball with your feet about hip width apart.
❚ Slowly walk your feet forward until you can lean back over the ball with your spine long, your legs straight, and your arms wide open (see figure).
❚ Enjoy several slow, steady breaths for 30 to 60 seconds.

Adjustments

If you feel challenged with balance for any reason (not enough sleep, not enough water, a rough day), you can move into this stretch with your knees bent. Bending the knees will allow you to feel more stable as you work toward straightening your legs in the future.

Lateral Stretch on Stability Ball

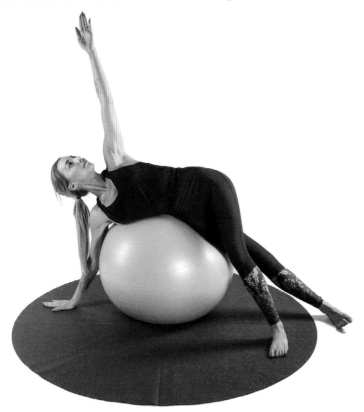

Benefits

This exercise stretches the entire length of the side of your body with focus on the waist muscles.

Feeling

In the practice of yoga, we speak a lot about the side body and breathing into its length. This refers to the feeling of support that the muscles on the sides of our bodies create when activated. Imagine that your oblique muscles are two pillars of strength that can help you stand tall with support from the inside out.

Instruction

- Begin kneeling next to a stability ball.
- Step your left foot slightly forward and lean onto the ball as you straighten both legs and place your right hand on the floor, with the left arm extended toward the sky. Your feet will be splayed (one about 12 to 24 inches in front of the other; see figure).
- Enjoy several slow, steady breaths for 30 to 60 seconds on each side.

Adjustments

If you feel like you need a little extra support with balance and stability, try practicing this stretch with your back foot up against the baseboard of a wall. Keeping your foot on the wall will help you stabilize the body.

Foam Roller for the Spine

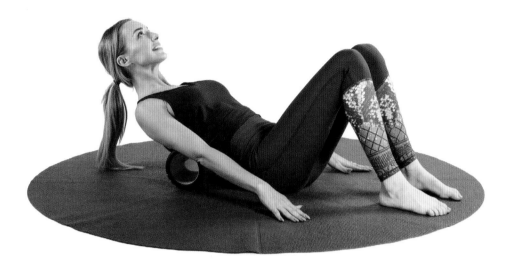

Benefits

This maneuver promotes myofascial release and feels really good on the muscles that support the spine, similar to the benefits of massage.

Feeling

Myofascial release involves placing pressure on the fascia, the body's connective tissue. This type of work is said to help reduce stress, work out adhesions, release tension, and improve circulation. Enjoy the pleasurable feeling of the pressure on your back body, similar to a massage therapist's hands pressing into your back.

Instruction

▌ Place the foam roller horizontally on your yoga mat.
▌ Lie down on top of the foam roller so that the lower back is supported by the foam roller with your feet approximately hip width apart, all ten toes pointed forward, and the knees tracking toward the second and third toes (see figure).
▌ Gently open your arms so that your fingers are supported by the floor.
▌ Begin to roll slowly up and down on the foam roller.

Adjustments

If you would like this gentle movement to feel more like a restorative yoga experience, consider diffusing eucalyptus oil in the room. This will instantly invite the feeling of a spalike experience as you open your sinuses while massaging your own back.

Supine Hand-to-Big-Toe Pose

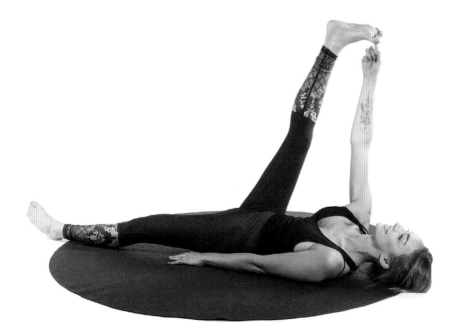

Benefits

This pose helps improve pelvic stability and increase flexibility in the lifted leg.

Feeling

There is a wonderful feeling of two lines of energy meeting and intersecting at the heart center. One line of energy is head to foot, and the other is side to side.

Instruction

- Lie faceup with your legs straight.
- Lift your right leg straight up to the sky with a strap, if used, wrapped around your right foot.
- Hold both ends of the strap, if used, in your right hand as you guide your right leg to the right.
- Make sure to keep the back of the left hip and the back of the left shoulder on the floor.
- Stretch out your left hand to the left and gently turn your head to gaze over your left middle finger.
- Enjoy several deep breaths, and then change sides.

Adjustments

This pose can be practiced with your first two fingers around your big toe if you are an advanced practitioner or if you have very long arms that easily reach to your feet (see figure). For beginners and after pregnancy, using a D-ring strap is a great way to make the action of reaching the foot effortless, so that you can focus on the shoulders and the back of the pelvis staying grounded.

Supine Hand-to-Big-Toe Pose With a Twist

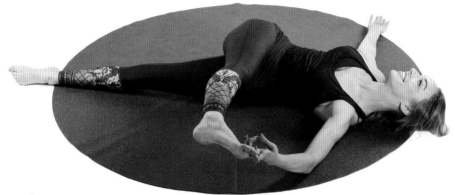

Benefits

This pose stretches the outer hip and thigh of the leg that is crossing the midline of the body. Twists are also said to help with digestion and elimination. While twists are contraindicated during pregnancy, they are safe now, especially since you are lying down and relaxed.

Feeling

Enjoy the feeling of twisting like a spiral from head to toe. This spiraling energy in the practice of yoga is called *kundalini energy*. Kundalini energy is said to be the energy of potential that lies dormant at the base of the spine and can be raised to the crown to tap into expanded states of consciousness. If this is brand new for you, imagine two spiraling columns of light dancing on either side of your spine, much like the double helix of DNA. Imagine those columns of light easily moving from the base of the spine up to your lower back and sacrum, gently rising to the midback, and then to the neck and the cervical spine. Envision this light easily expanding up to the crown of your head and beyond.

Instruction

- Lie faceup with your legs straight.
- Lift your right leg straight up to the sky with a strap, if used, wrapped around your right foot.
- Hold both ends of the strap in your left hand as you guide your right leg across your body to the left.
- Keep the back of both of your shoulders down on the floor.
- Work toward gently guiding the right hip down so as to lengthen the right side of your waist.
- Take your gaze to the right so that your head and neck continue the energy of the spiral through the cervical spine.

Adjustments

This pose can be practiced with your first two fingers around your big toe if you are an advanced practitioner or if you have very long arms that easily reach to your feet (see figure). For beginners and after pregnancy, using a D-ring strap is a great way to make the action of reaching the foot effortless. You can deepen the twist by bending the bottom knee and taking the opposite hand to the foot. From above, the body will look a bit like a pinwheel.

Putting It All Together

Two sample recovery yoga practices are included here to start you back on the road to core strength recovery. Remember to take your time and listen to your body. The Dear Mama: Gentle Recovery Practice is a great place to ease your body back into a gentle yoga practice. To reinvigorate your core muscles, try the Wake Me Up: Deep Core Recovery Practice. Your core muscles are known as your powerhouse muscles in the world of Pilates, and with good reason. The core helps power many of our daily activities as moms, including lifting your baby, and putting her in the crib at night. Rebuilding the strength and harmony of your core muscles does not happen overnight, and a gentle, balanced, and focused workout goes a long way with postpartum recovery.

DEAR MAMA: GENTLE RECOVERY YOGA PRACTICE

This is an exciting time in life, right after you've had a baby. Your body, mind, and heart are forever changed. Your doctor will clear you for exercise at around four to six weeks after labor and delivery (sometimes longer for C-section). This practice is designed to be a gentle reentry into flow classes and practices and to help you open up the front body, meaning that as we stretch into gentle backbends supported on a stability ball, there is space to take a deep breath and stretch. Many moms find that their posture has changed from the Donald Duck style swayback of pregnancy into hunching over into what I politely call *baby adoring pose*. Think about it: If you are constantly leaning over to nurse or bottle-feed your baby, to change diapers, to push a stroller, and to enjoy sweet gazes at your baby's face, then stretching in the opposite direction is good, smart movement. We want to stretch the chest and the front of the shoulders in addition to lengthening the torso and feeling a satisfying stretch in the whole front side of your body.

Exercise	Page	Focus	Reps/Time
Child's Pose	59	Stretches lower back and hips; invites ease	3-5 slow, deep, centering breaths focusing on the inhalation and the exhalation being equal in length
Easy Pose	41	Gently stretches thighs; invites ease	3 breaths in Easy Pose
Unicorn and Rainbow Pose	42	Lower back and abdomen	5 rounds (it is OK to gently tuck the tailbone now that you are postnatal)
Down Dog Into Stacked Hip Variation	162	Lower back, hamstrings, calves	3 breaths in Down Dog Pose; 3 breaths with the right leg up; 3 breaths with the left leg up
Standing Lateral Stretch	106	Legs, core, triceps, shoulders	3 breaths in Mountain Pose; 3 breaths leaning to the right; 3 breaths leaning to the left

Exercise	Page	Focus	Reps/Time
Half Sun Salutation With Backbend	163	Shoulders, core strength, flexibility	3 rounds of Half Sun Salutation; remember that each movement corresponds to an inhalation or exhalation
Supported Backbend on Stability Ball	164	Abdomen, chest	5-7 deep breaths
Lateral Stretch on Stability Ball	165	Triceps, obliques, outer thighs	5 deep breaths on the right and the left
Foam Roller for the Spine	166	Muscles that support the spine	60-90 seconds on your back
Supine Hand-to-Big-Toe Pose	167	Hamstrings	5-9 breaths on the right and left
Supine Hand-to-Big-Toe Pose With a Twist	168	Outer thighs and hips	5-9 breaths on the right and left
Deep Relaxation Pose	66	Entire body	1-3 minutes

WAKE ME UP: DEEP CORE RECOVERY PRACTICE

Your life slowly begins to establish a new rhythm when your baby is around eight weeks old. As your energy levels return and you emerge from the foggy bliss of labor and delivery, waking up the deeper core muscles can feel really good. This practice will reawaken your core stabilizers in a safe and mindful way. Remembering how to engage your abs, strengthen your obliques, and stabilize your trunk (less sexy word for core) can begin to empower you with strength from the inside out, creating a strong foundation on which you can build in future months.

This too is good, smart work that will help to draw everything back to the midline. This simply means that for 40 weeks your body was working to expand and create space for baby but now is the time to start bringing it all back in the direction of your center. It is important to remember to build on a strong foundation of strength rather than jumping directly back into full range of motion leg lifts to train your abs, so start with deep, targeted abdominal work like the exercises in this practice. Note that all of the exercises in this practice are included in many physical therapy protocols for DR. Use this practice at around six to eight weeks postpartum, with doctor's clearance.

Exercise	Page	Focus	Reps/Time
Isometric Abdominal Contraction	153	TVA and abs	Contract for 20 seconds as you breathe deeply; emphasize the exhalation as you contract; do 2 sets of 3 reps
Bent-Knee Fallout	154	TVA and abs	2 sets of 10 reps, alternating right and left
Bridge Pose	155	Lower back, glutes, hamstrings	2 sets of 10 reps, holding for 10 seconds each
Unilateral Isometric Hip Flexion	156	TVA, abs, psoas	1 set of 10 reps each to the right and left
Arm-Only Pointer Dog Pose	157	Core stabilization	3-5 deep breaths on the right; pause in the center to find balance; and then 3-5 deep breaths on the left

Exercise	Page	Focus	Reps/Time
Prone Bent-Knee Lift	158	Hamstrings, glutes	2 sets of 10 reps
Heel Squeeze	159	Thighs, glutes, pelvic stabilization and strength	1 set of 10 reps, holding for 10 seconds each
Straight-Leg Raise	160	External rotators of the hips, glutes, lower back	2 sets of 10 reps to the right and left
Pointer Dog Pose	43	Core stabilization	3-5 deep breaths on the right; pause in the center to find balance; and then 3-5 deep breaths on the left
Forearm Plank Pose	161	TVA, abs, lower back, obliques, shoulder stabilizers	2 sets of 20-second holds
Deep Relaxation Pose	66	Entire body	3-5 minutes

*M*ommy Move

Diaphragmatic Breathing

After the first 72 hours of labor and delivery, you will probably be at home with your beautiful baby. Breathing into your belly a few times can feel really good and help to bring more oxygen into your body while you are healing. Diaphragmatic breathing is called *ujjayi pranayama*, which means victorious breath. Enjoy a slow, steady inhalation through the nose that creates a little whispery sound as you close the glottis (back of the throat) to gently vibrate. This is very different from sniffing, as you will be inhaling with your diaphragm moving down, leading to the feeling of filling the belly with breath. On your exhalation, exhale through the nose only as you envision the diaphragm floating up, helping you to release the air. This release of air through your nose will cause your abdominal muscles to gently contract. This is not intended to be a workout; on the contrary, it is more about inviting the energy of healing and restoration.

During pregnancy, it is common to daydream of being able to lie on your belly again. Surprisingly, it does not feel that good after you have given birth. Your breasts are engorged and tender so lying on the belly can be quite uncomfortable for a few more weeks. Breathing into the belly will give you a sweet feeling of connection with your diaphragm without overexerting yourself, and it can be practiced lying down on your back or sitting up.

*I*nformation No One Tells You

Disposable Underwear

The pelvic floor acts as a hammock of sorts, helping to support the weight of your organs. During pregnancy, the strain on this muscle group is increased because of the weight of the growing baby in your uterus. After baby is born, these muscles are healing. (If you had an episiotomy, additional healing time might be needed.) All of these factors can lead to what many politely call the pee sneeze. This is a lighthearted reference to the fact that you might experience LBL. Such leakage can increase when there is downward pressure on the pelvic floor from a sneeze, a cough, or a belly laugh. Also, right after you have a baby, there is some blood, similar to a light menstrual flow, called *lochia*. Both the lochia and the light bladder leakage can ruin your undergarments. Using disposable underwear can save you money because you won't need to throw away all your undies.

If you're wondering if you need disposable undies if you had a C-section, the answer is yes. You still carried the weight of your baby on the pelvic floor, so there will be some bleeding.

*L*ove-Your-Baby Visualization

Synchronizing Your Breathing With Baby

You can do this meditation any time you choose, including while nursing. While holding your baby, begin to count the length of your inhalation. Try to stretch the duration of the inhalation to about five or six seconds. Now, do the same with the exhalation. Continue to silently count the length of your breathing cycle until it is slow, steady, and consistent. Now, close your eyes and start to feel your baby's breath cycle. It will naturally be shorter because its lungs are smaller. Notice how baby is breathing. Throughout this practice, stay mindful of keeping your breathing steady. You are modeling a full deep breath for your baby. When we breathe slowly and fully, a wonderful thing often happens: Baby begins to mirror this breathing pattern. Again, baby's breathing will always be a little quicker, but it can feel your sense of calm and peace. This is like a salve to the nervous system; when practiced regularly, it is something you can call on when needed. For example, if you are on an airplane with a baby who is overstimulated, you can come back to this calming, centering breath and, feeling your peace, your baby can begin to settle.

*F*un Foods

In many cultures around the world, women enjoy a sweet time after labor and delivery in the comfort of their own homes, very often being taken care of by female family members. In India, for the first forty days of the postpartum period new mothers are often cared for by their own mothers and their sisters with warm sesame oil massages and foods that are said to calm the air (*vata*) element in the body (*vata* and the *doshas* are covered more extensively in chapter 2). Almond milk is a nourishing postpartum drink that is also said to help with lactation.

Almond Milk

> 1/4 cup almonds
>
> 1 cup of milk, warmed to desired temperature
>
> 1/2 teaspoon clarified butter (ghee)
>
> 1 teaspoon maple syrup

Soak the almonds for 8 to 10 hours in water at room temperature. When ready, slip the skin from the almonds. Combine with the remaining ingredients in blender. Blend until smooth. Serve warm.

Yield: *1 serving*

Mommy and Me

Practicing yoga with your baby can be a sweet way to bond with your little one while you regain and reclaim your physical strength. For 40 weeks or so, your body had a roommate and needed to make space to accommodate your little one. Now that your baby is in your arms and not in your belly, it can be really fun to exercise with your baby. But it can be challenging to leave your baby at home while you go to exercise, and leaving your baby with a caretaker to go take a class can pull on your heartstrings, not to mention your bank account.

When my older son, Cruz, was born, I spent a lot of time discovering different parenting styles. I quickly learned that the decision of how to parent was not just up to me; it was up to him, too. He let me know very clearly that attachment parenting was his preferred method, and he spent most of his first two years of life snuggled on my shoulder, so it was important to find ways that I could exercise with him. Walking with a carrier, practicing yoga, and attending mommy-and-me swim classes were all effective ways for us to play together while I rebuilt my strength, and he gained his own head and neck strength.

The tremendous amount of physical training that babies do all day helps them gain the natural curves in their spine. When your baby starts to lift her head and neck, she is gaining the curve in her cervical spine. When she starts to push up into a position similar to locust and cobra pose, she is gaining the curve in her lumbar spine, which will allow her to crawl and eventually walk. Additionally, when she is lying on the changing table and starts to lift her head and feet, she is effectively training her abdominal muscles. Babies are natural yogis and the Oh Baby practice that accompanies this chapter is inspired by the same types of training that your baby practices all day. As with any type of training for you, it is important to have your doctor's clearance, as discussed in chapter 8.

Safe Grip

During mommy-and-me yoga practice, it is important to hold your baby with both arms at all times for safety. If your baby is a newborn, I would recommend letting it lie down in whatever position it is most comfortable: in a baby papasan, in a Moses basket, or swaddled on your yoga mat. Once baby starts to gain head and neck control, it's a good time to start to hold it while you do some of the standing poses. Younger babies often prefer heart-to-heart holding, meaning that your baby is cradled in your arms facing in toward your chest. Babies over six months of age often prefer to have their spine to your heart, so they can look out toward the world and their surroundings while still feeling the warmth and safety of mommy. Whichever way your baby is facing, remember to hold your baby with both of your arms. For older babies, you can place one of your forearms under your baby's bottom and your other forearm around the abdomen. I cue this in class by saying "Use your safe grip, which is one forearm under tushie, other forearm around tummy" (see figure 9.1).

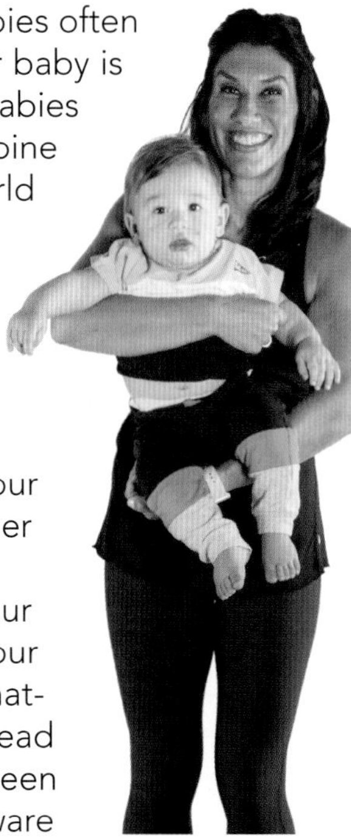

Figure 9.1 Safe grip.

For your wrist health, it is important to keep your wrists neutral or almost neutral while holding your baby. Holding the wrist in a flexed position is a natural default position for many moms, but it can lead to tremendous strain and pain in the wrists. (I've seen a lot of moms with wrist braces as a result.) Be aware of the position of your hands and try to allow them to be a natural extension of your forearms. If your wrists are already strained, you might choose to use a front carrier to hold your baby while you enjoy certain movements like squats. If you are using a front carrier for exercise, I recommend one that allows your baby to sit at the center of your torso, rather than a sling. Slings are not secure enough for certain movements, and it is important that you can always see your baby's face during any type of exercise together. Front carriers work very well for walking; many moms refer to this as *wearing your baby*. This idea has been around for centuries. Many indigenous cultures enjoy baby wearing. Baby wearing seems to have taken a dip in popularity in the early 1900s, when carriages came into fashion in England. In the United States, wearing your baby has gained popularity in the last 20 years, and studies show that babies who are carried tend to cry less.

Proper Lifting Mechanics

Each time you lift your baby, you are lifting weight. Many times, you lift even more than your baby's weight throughout a normal day. For example, if your baby weighs 20 pounds and is in a 22-pound car seat, that means that every time you lift your baby while it's in the car seat, you have to lift 42 pounds! To take the example further, you may then need to put the car seat with your baby in the snap-in stroller. In this simple example from daily life, you have had to lift 42 pounds several times, and you may experience some twisting of your torso as you take a heavy stroller out of the car or remove the car seat from the car. Twisting or rotating while carrying weight creates torque. Torque on the spine can lead to injury and pain, so remember to turn your feet, hips, and shoulders toward the object you are lifting to reduce the risk of injury.

Each time you lift weight, whether it is at the gym or lifting your beautiful baby, it is important to use proper lifting mechanics. Pain in the lower back can be a result of poor mechanics in daily activities with your baby. Practice these simple steps to avoid "mommy back" and keep your lower back healthy and happy.

- Bend your knees every time you lift your baby from the floor.
- When lifting your baby or the car seat (or both) out of the car, turn to face baby rather than facing the back of the vehicle and then twisting your torso.
- When carrying your baby, alternate which side of your chest, or which hip, baby is close to.
- Relax your shoulders down and back, rather than slumping forward or shrugging.
- When lifting baby or any other weight, keep your pelvis underneath your torso rather than pushing your pelvis forward to compensate for the weight.
- Engage your core muscles every time you lift.
- It can be helpful to exhale as you initially lift.

The most common places you will be lifting your baby from are usually the floor, the crib, the changing table, and the car. Each of these is a unique scenario that has its own requirements.

Floor

When lifting your baby from the floor, make sure you have good traction on your feet, whether it is an athletic shoe or a grippy sock. Bend your knees generously and squat so that you can use the strength of your lower body to lift. Never move from sitting to standing while holding your baby in the tub. Instead, call for a family member to come take the baby when you are ready to exit the tub. See figure 9.2 for an example of how to properly lift your baby from the floor.

Crib or Playpen

Depending on the height of the crib or playpen and the age of your baby, the mattress might be quite low and the railing fairly high. If this is the case, consider purchasing a sturdy stepping stool that is wide, with a solid foundation. Place the stool next to the crib or playpen so that you don't have to try to hoist your torso over the side of the crib. If possible, bend your knees a bit and engage your core as you lift your baby. See figure 9.3 for an example of how to properly lift your baby from the playpen or crib.

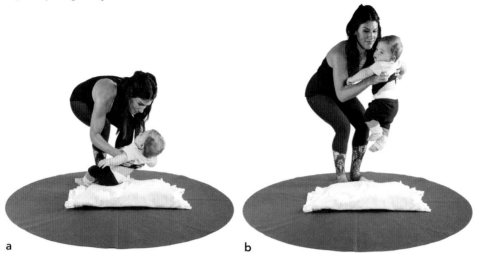

Figure 9.2 Lifting your baby from the floor.

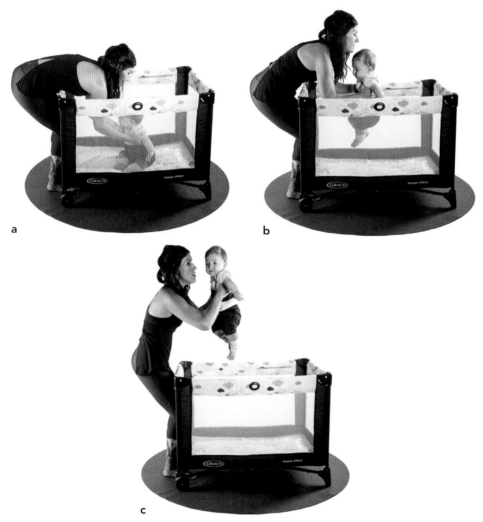

Figure 9.3 Lifting your baby from the playpen or crib.

Changing Table

Baby should always be secured with the safety belt on an elevated changing table. When lifting baby from the table, move slowly and mindfully as you first lift and then turn away from the table. Too often, this is done in one movement, creating torque on the spine.

Car

When you lift your baby from the car, bend your knees and engage your core. Again, lift baby first and then turn your body out of the car, rather than doing it in one movement, especially if you are lifting baby right in the car seat. See figure 9.4 for an example of how to properly lift your baby from the car or stroller.

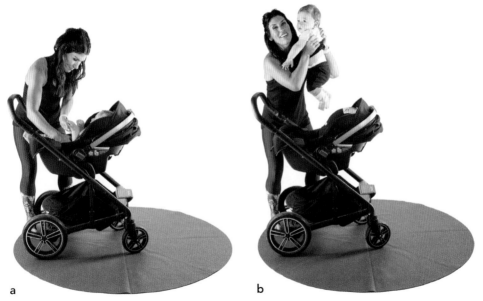

a   b

Figure 9.4   Lifting your baby from the car or stroller.

Baby Yoga

If you practice yoga in a studio setting, your pediatrician might also want you to wait until your baby receives a particular vaccine before going to public areas. At home, you can usually begin practicing with a very young baby simply lying at the front of your yoga mat.

Younger babies usually enjoy lying at the front of your yoga mat on a cozy blanket. If you know your baby likes to be swaddled, you can wrap it in the swaddling blanket. If baby is asleep in an infant seat or a baby papasan, it is totally fine to leave that at the front of the mat so you can watch baby while you enjoy your yoga practice. But be aware that it is not recommended to have baby spend long periods of time in the car seat. Baby's spine is still

Staying Safe

During your baby's first year, there are some safety guidelines to remember when practicing yoga with your baby.

■ Baby should be in cool, comfortable clothing.

■ Use a safe grip to hold your baby, or a front carrier (not a sling).

■ Room should be a comfortable temperature, at or near 72 degrees.

■ Work on a stable and dry surface to avoid slipping.

■ Keep all toys off your mat to avoid tripping.

■ No prone work (on the tummy) for baby right after eating (e.g., Flying Baby exercise).

■ If baby stiffens a limb, do not try to pull or work through it.

developing, and prolonged periods in the car seat (or any seat) are not good for the development of your baby's spine. Many manufacturers abide by the rule stating that your baby should not be in a car seat for more than two hours within any 24-hour period.

Around four or five months old, babies start to explore tummy time and roll onto their tummy while you practice. Around eight or nine months old, your baby will probably start to model some of the movements that you do in your yoga practice. She might start to reach up or down, or anticipate you giving her a kiss every time she sees you in Plank Pose. This rapid development is amazing to witness, and by the time that your baby is about 12 to 14 months old, chances are he will have mastered Up Dog and Down Dog, will often roll over into Cobra, or lie on his back and do Happy Baby Pose. You can help baby do some simple exercises in an interactive form of play. As an adult, you may find that you develop a higher level of body awareness through movement and yoga poses. You can encourage the same awareness in your baby as you spend time together on your mat. Here are some ideas for games that you can play together during your yoga practice, and which are specifically intended to benefit your baby.

■ *Play-peek-a-boo.* This teaches your baby the idea of object permanence, even when she cannot see you momentarily. You are still there, and she will start to learn that.

■ *Sing "Head, shoulders, knees, and toes."* As you sing, touch the relevant part of your baby so that he can start to learn the names of body parts.

- *Give a gentle tummy massage.* Make very light clockwise circles with your fingers on your baby's tummy. This can help to promote digestion and alleviate gas.
- *Gentle bicycles.* Very gently bicycle your baby's legs, which can also help to alleviate gas.
- *Cross-patterning.* Touch your baby's right hand to her left foot a few times, and then switch to the other side. This helps stimulate the part of the brain responsible for reading.
- *Sing to your baby.* Pick songs like "Twinkle, Twinkle Little Star," and "The Itsy Bitsy Spider," which incorporate hand movements.

Yoga Poses and Exercises with Your Baby

After your baby is born, your body will need to work in a different way than when you were pregnant. During pregnancy, your core held your baby. Now you can hold your baby in your arms and use the power in your lower body when lifting and lowering your baby. Your core will still be an integral part of lifting your baby, but now it is safe to draw your core in and up, and feel the support of the corsetlike muscles inside. The following exercises are recommended to enjoy with your baby. They are a form of functional training; they will help you with proper lifting mechanics and to gain the strength to continue to lift your baby comfortably as baby grows.

Mommy-and-Me with a Toddler

Try these fun, simple movements that are very similar to common yoga poses.

- Reach up to touch the stars.
- Bend forward and tickle your toes.
- Step back to Down Dog and bark like a puppy.
- Bring your tummy to the floor in Cobra Pose and hiss like a snake.
- Come to your hands and knees and look up to the sky as you moo like a cow, then round your spine as you meow like a cat.
- Come into Child's Pose and play the quiet game for 10 seconds.
- Repeat the sequence as many times as your toddler enjoys it.

If you have an infant also, let your infant watch you and your toddler as you practice yoga together. Your baby might giggle or smile as they watch their older sibling and hear the animal noises.

Mommy-and-Me Sun Salutation A

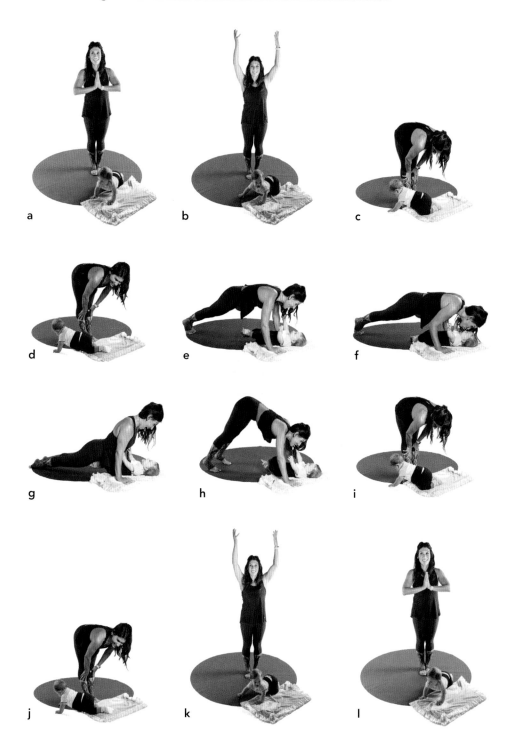

Benefits

This sequence warms the entire body.

Feeling

Invite the warmth and radiance of sunlight. Feel that your body is warming up from the inside out, and that your inner light is expanding with each inhalation as you let go of stress and tension with every exhalation. Also, remember to invite the spirit of play with your baby. You can blow kisses, giggle, wink, or whatever you know will make your baby smile and giggle with delight.

Instruction

- Begin standing in Mountain Pose, with your feet together and your hands in namaste (see figure a).
- Inhale and lift your arms straight up to the sky (see figure b).
- Exhale and fold forward, bringing your hands onto both lower legs and your nose toward your knees. This is a sweet opportunity to tickle your baby's toes or tummy (see figure c).
- Inhale and rise up halfway (see figure d); exhale and step back to Plank Pose. Stay in Plank for your inhalation (see figure e).
- Exhale and move through Chaturanga, which is like Plank, but with bent elbows pointed straight back (it is the bottom of a triceps push-up). Keeping your abdomen hovering above the floor, you can kiss your baby's nose (see figure f).
- Inhale and lift your heart to the sky for Cobra Pose (see figure g).
- Exhale and return to Down Dog (see figure h).
- Stay in Down Dog for three to five deep breaths.
- Step or jump your feet to your hands into a deep Forward Fold (see figure i).
- Inhale and come up halfway, with your head reaching forward and your tailbone reaching back (see figure j).
- Exhale and subside into deep Forward Fold again.
- Inhale and rise to standing with your arms reaching to the sky (see figure k).
- Exhale and return to Mountain Pose with your hands at your heart (see figure l).

Adjustments

If Plank and Chaturanga feel very challenging with your knees above the floor, you can practice both movements with your knees on your mat. You can also place a folded blanket under your knees so that you have some padding.

Kiss-the-Baby Chaturanga Pose

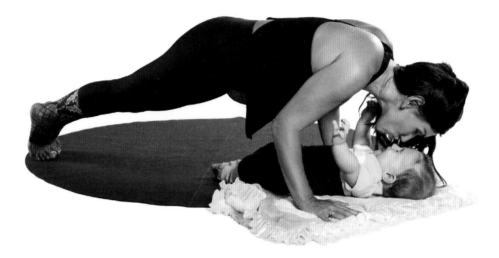

Benefits

This pose strengthens the upper body as well as the core stabilizers.

Feeling

Traditionally this pose is practiced as part of a Sun Salutation, and the feeling is that of great control. As you slowly lower, use your strength to gauge the speed at which you lower. This variation, created by Mothers Into Living Fit, is much more fun because you have a moment of sweet connection with your baby at the same time as you are staying dedicated to your strength.

Instruction

▮ Begin in Plank Pose with your hands directly underneath your shoulders, so your shoulder, elbow, and wrist joints are aligned.

▮ Feel the strength in your core, making sure that you are neither dipping down in the lower back nor lifting the hips.

▮ Slowly bend your elbows, taking care that your elbows point straight back toward your feet and not out to the sides of the room. (This is different from a traditional push-up, in which your elbows point outward). Making sure you maintain your torso hovering above the floor, kiss your baby (see figure).

▮ Traditionally, you will transition from here into Cobra or Up Dog. Take care not to collapse out of the pose; instead, lower slowly and with control.

Adjustments

You can practice this movement on your knees to take some of the weight off your upper body. If you choose to practice on your knees (which is fantastic for beginners and for those regaining their strength), you may want to place a folded blanket under your knees for added cushion.

Squat With Baby

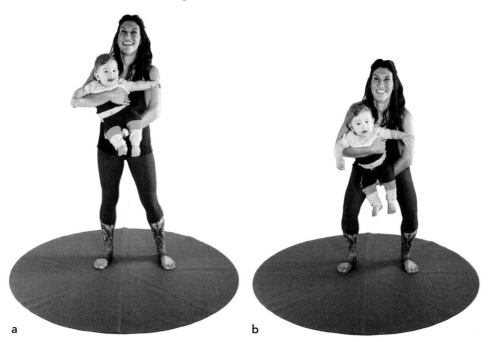

a   b

Benefits

This exercise strengthens your lower body, upper body, and core.

Feeling

Feel the strength of your lower body driving the power of this movement. This is a functional movement, simply meaning that squatting is the correct way to pick babies up from the floor or from a car seat on the floor. Bending your knees supports your lower back, and by using correct lifting mechanics you can keep your lower back happy and healthy.

Instruction

- Stand with your feet hip width apart and all ten toes pointing straight forward.
- Hold your baby with a safe grip: one forearm under baby's tushie and the other forearm in front of baby's tummy (see figure a). Note that this instruction is for babies with head and neck control.
- As you inhale, begin to bend your knees with your hips moving back as though you were going to sit in a chair. Make sure to stand up tall in the upper body so that you are not leaning forward (see figure b).
- As you exhale, slowly straighten the legs and feel the power in your thighs and glutes.

Adjustments

You can perform this exercise in front of a mirror with your baby facing the mirror. The mirror will allow you visual feedback on your own form, ensuring that you are performing the exercise correctly. Besides, babies often think the baby in the mirror is another baby and they will giggle and smile with glee as they see the baby in the mirror smiling back.

Lunge With Baby

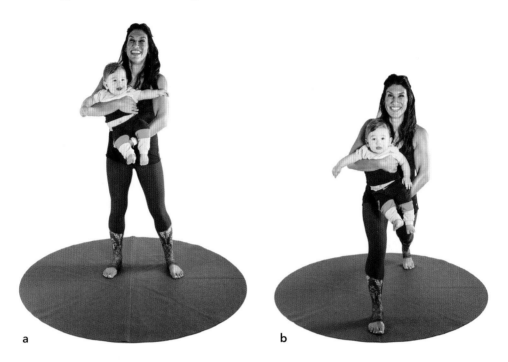

a   b

Benefits

This exercise strengthens the quads, hamstrings, core, and biceps.

Feeling

Connect to the feeling of moving straight up and down as opposed to forward and back. To visualize this, think of the movement like a merry-go-round. Children giggle with glee as the horses move up and down, and will often do the same as mommy moves up and down.

Instruction

- Begin standing upright with your core engaged and your baby in a safe and comfortable position for both you and your baby (see figure a).
- Step your right foot forward and bend your right knee to a 90 degree angle (see figure b) with your back knee almost touching the floor at the end of the forward movement.
- Slowly rise and straighten your front leg on the exhalation.
- Repeat the exercise for the desired number of repetitions on the right and the left sides. Remember to breathe deeply and to straighten the front leg on the exhalation, and inhale as you bend the front knee.

Adjustments

Younger babies who do not have head and neck control should be held in your arms against your chest. Older babies often like to face out (away from your face) so they can see the world around them while in the safety of your arms. You can use a safe grip with your baby facing out, or hold your baby seated on your front thigh.

Shoulder Press With Baby

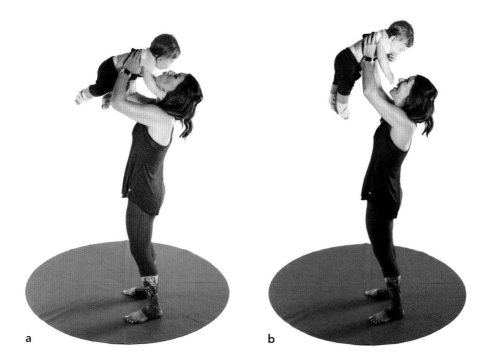

a   b

Benefits

This exercise helps strengthen the shoulders, biceps, and core stabilizers.

Feeling

Feel the strength in your upper body as you lift your baby up toward the sky. This is a functional movement; there will always be occasions when you need to lift baby. Have fun with this movement and let the little kiss you give your baby at the bottom of the movement become your incentive and inspiration to continue doing more repetitions. Your baby's smile is the sweetest reward for a job well done.

Instruction

- Stand with your feet hip width apart and a slight bend in your knees.
- Hold your baby around the torso with both your hands (see figure a). Note that this exercise is intended to enjoy with babies who have head and neck control.
- Slowly exhale and begin to lift your baby up to a height that you can comfortably control, using the strength of your upper body (see figure b).
- Inhale and bring baby back down toward your face, smiling at your baby each time.

Adjustments

You can give your baby a kiss every time you lower it toward your face. You can also choose to alternate kissing each cheek: gently lift baby up in the air, and as she comes close to your face, kiss her right cheek; lift baby up again, and this time as she comes close to your face, kiss her left cheek.

Boat Pose With Baby

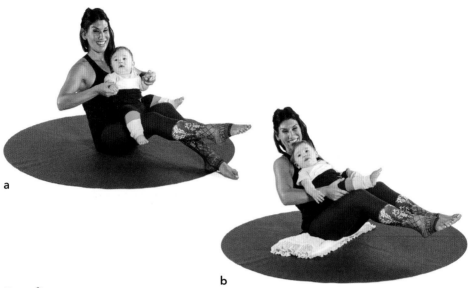

a

b

Benefits

This pose strengthens the core and the psoas. It also helps secondary muscles, including the shoulders and biceps, depending on how you hold your baby.

Feeling

Feel the strength in your deep abdominal muscles as you play and sing. It is interesting to note that Paramahansa Yogananda, one of the yogis who helped bring yoga to the West, refers to "Row, Row, Row Your Boat" in his teachings. He taught that mortal life is a dream, and that the concept of "life is but a dream" is a deeply mystical thought.

Instruction

- Begin seated on the floor with your baby in your lap. For younger babies, you can cradle baby in your arms. For babies with head and neck control, have your baby's spine against your torso (see figure a). Wrap your arms around baby so that he feels secure in your arms, and make sure not to flex your wrists. A slight bend is OK, but remember not to have a deep bend at the wrist crease.
- Slowly lean your torso back toward a 45 degree angle. It's OK to stay a little bit higher than this, especially if this is a new movement for you. Lift your legs and feel the strength in your core (see figure b).
- Breathe deeply, and if you choose, you can sing "Row, Row, Row Your Boat" to your baby.

Adjustments

If the pose is too challenging with the legs straight, you can bend your knees to make it a little bit easier. You can also "rock the boat" a little if you would like to increase the physical challenge; simply lower your upper and lower body slightly, and then lift again, in a rhythmic, rocking motion. Note that this is not an appropriate pose if you have DR.

Flying Baby

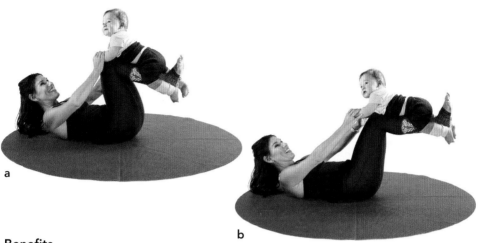

a

b

Benefits

This maneuver strengthens the core and the psoas.

Feeling

Playtime! Mommy is baby's first playground; your body becomes a jungle gym for your baby. Connect to the feeling of strength, and the structure of your body providing a safe space for your baby to play and "fly."

Instruction

- Begin sitting up with your knees bent and feet on the floor. Gently bring your baby to a standing position while holding the forearms securely with your hands. Note that this exercise is intended for babies who have head and neck control.
- Lie back slowly and let your baby lie on your shins (see figure a). Lift your head, neck, and shoulders off the floor as you engage your abdominal muscles. Inhale and let your legs slide forward a few inches, ensuring that you can maintain a safe grip around your baby's forearms (see figure b).
- Exhale and draw your knees toward you to feel the contraction in your core muscles.
- Repeat. You can sing to your baby throughout the movement if you like. After you finish the exercise, you can either lower your baby onto your abdomen and chest or rock yourself up to return to the starting position.

Adjustments

If your baby does not yet have head and neck control, you can perform the exercise with baby lying down next to you. In this case, you can support your head and neck with your hands behind your head. If you are performing the exercise with your baby on your shins and experience any pain in your head and neck, you can do the exercise with your head on the ground. The cue that is given in most fitness classes regarding crunches applies here: Pretend that you have a tomato under your chin when you lift the head and neck, so that you do not tuck the chin. This will help you to maintain a neutral cervical spine and avoid pain. Note that this exercise should be done at least 45 minutes after your baby's last meal to avoid an upset tummy.

Kneeling Sun Salutation With Baby

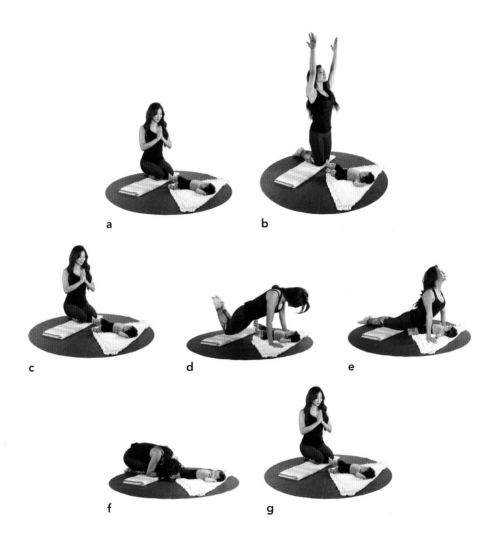

Benefits

A more gentle variation of the Sun Salutations, this sequence warms the entire body.

Feeling

As in all Sun Salutations, there is a feeling of welcoming the possibilities of the new day and of this new phase of life with your baby. At the same time, you have an opportunity to check in with your constant companion, your breath. Feel the reassuring nature of the constancy of the breath while you invite the new possibilities and celebrate the changes that have come with becoming a mother.

Instruction

- Place baby at the top of your mat and begin in Hero Pose with your knees together and your hands at your heart (see figure a).
- Inhale and lift up tall on your knees so that your hips are directly over your knees and your arms are reaching to the sky (see figure b).
- Exhale and return to Hero Pose with your hands at your heart. Stay here for your next inhale (see figure c).
- Exhale and shift forward to Modified Plank with your knees on the floor (see figure d).
- Inhale and glide your abdomen and chest forward into Cobra Pose with the heart lifting and a long, graceful neck with the trapezius muscles relaxed, not shrugged (see figure e).
- Inhale and bring your knees gently onto the floor. Exhale and glide your hips back to sit onto your heels into Child's Pose (see figure f).
- Inhale and return to Hero Pose with the hands at the heart center (see figure g).

Adjustments

A folded blanket under your knees can provide cushion, especially if you are working with a thin yoga mat. This is a great choice of Sun Salutation variation for anyone beginning to reclaim their strength, especially new moms.

Easy Twist With Baby

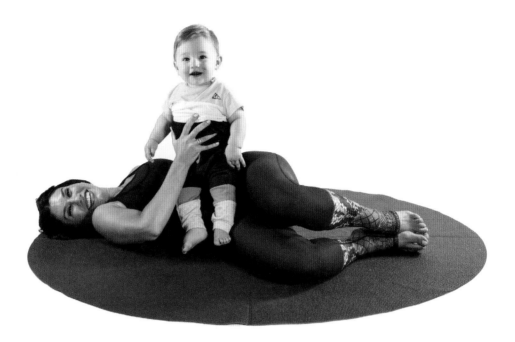

Benefits

This exercise releases tension in the back.

Feeling

Let all tension in your body, mind, and heart release with each breath. By having your baby sit on your top hip, your baby's weight will naturally give you a similar adjustment that a yoga teacher would give you.

Instruction

- Lie down on your back and pull your knees in to your chest.
- On your exhalation, swivel your knees to the right until the outer right thigh touches the floor. If baby has head and neck control, he can sit on your top hip or rest on your chest.
- Repeat on the other side.

Hero Pose

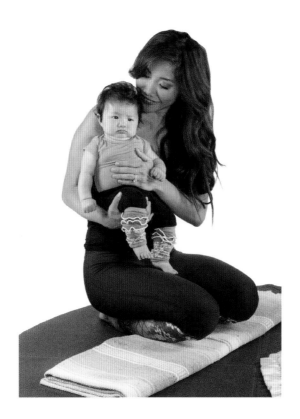

Benefits

This pose stretches the hips and the groin and elongates the front of the body.

Feeling

You are heroic. Strong. Feel the power in your body and celebrate the superhero-like strength you have as a woman. You are a hero to your baby, and you have great reservoirs of power you can draw from. Allow yourself to be still, breathe deeply, and know that you can rise to any challenge.

Instruction

- Begin seated back on your knees, with the knees together (see figure).
- Be aware that the feet are softly resting straight back on the floor and not sickling (that is, try not to roll to the outer arch of the foot, especially if you know that you have a tendency to supinate, or if you wear orthotics).
- Bring the hands to the heart and breathe slowly and deeply or hold your baby.

Fish Pose

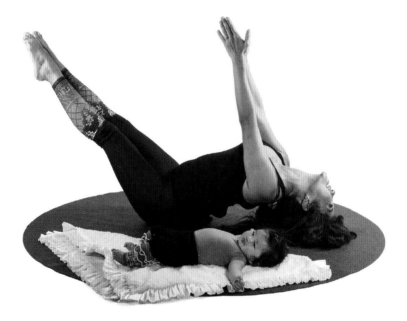

Benefits

This pose stretches the front of the body, especially the chest, shoulders, and throat.

Feeling

Lift the heart to the sky as though your chest were the fin on a fish's back; the heart steers your course toward love. You can close your eyes and take a few moments to reflect on the new waters you are navigating as a mother and as a woman. Let your heart lead the way.

Instruction

- Begin lying flat on your back.
- Lift your legs straight up toward the sky with all ten toes pointing up, so that the legs are slightly rotated inward. Lift your sternum to the sky and slide your head back under you until you can gently rest on the crown of your head (see figure).
- Breathe deeply and enjoy the stretch through the front of the body as you activate and strengthen your midback or posture muscles.

Adjustments

This pose can be made easier by resting a block underneath your midback to create a passive or restorative variation of Fish Pose. Or you can make the pose harder by crossing your legs into full Lotus Position, if that is available to you (that is, if your hips are flexible and you regularly practice lotus). In either variation, make sure that you take care to find a comfortable angle for your head and neck. The depth of this pose is largely dictated by the flexibility of the midback and chest, in addition to the neck. Be gentle and approach the pose slowly and gently.

Fitness Fun at the Playground

When your baby is old enough to go to a local park or playground, you can start to add fun movements incorporating the playground equipment. Here are some quick and easy ideas to get you started.

Babies in Strollers

If your baby has head and neck control, place your baby in the baby-friendly swing and stand at the front of the swing. Each time you gently push the swing, do an Alternating Reverse Lunge.

Crawling Babies

If your baby is crawling into the sandbox, sit alongside the sandbox edge and lean back with your upper body as you keep your feet planted in the sand. Try to maintain this position for at least 20 seconds in an isometric contraction of the abdominal muscles. It's very similar to the Boat Pose in yoga.

Toddlers

If your baby is walking and ready for a seesaw, you can move the opposite end of the seesaw up and down with your hands. Each time you push down with your hands, contract your triceps, and let this become a triceps pushdown.

Young Children

Use the monkey bars with your children. It provides an opportunity to improve upper body strength as you challenge yourself to swing from rung to rung. You can also hang from the bars and lift your knees for reps. This will help to train both your upper body strength and your core strength.

Here are some other ideas for exercises you can do at the park when your baby or toddler is lying or playing next to you.

- Pull-ups on the parallel bars
- Push-ups with your hands on a park bench
- Triceps dips with your hands on a park bench
- Squats: Repeat a seated-to-standing position as many times as you can in one minute
- Step-ups onto a park bench
- Leg abduction with one foot on a park bench
- Calf raises with your hands on the side of any structure

Putting It All Together

If you have a set schedule for your workouts with your baby, you'll have something tangible to keep you on track so that you are training in a balanced way, incorporating all the elements of fitness (strength training, flexibility training, and cardiovascular training). I suggest starting off with walking and baby wearing the first week that you have your doctor's clearance for exercise. If that goes well and you are feeling great, you can introduce the Baby Love and Oh Baby practices. Ultimately, I suggest you walk 20 minutes three times a week and alternate between the Baby Love and Oh Baby practices on the other four days.

BABY LOVE: POSTNATAL PRACTICE

Bonding with your baby and smiling at your little one while you are reclaiming your strength is a lot of fun. This practice is intended for those who are at least eight weeks postpartum; it builds slowly with a few challenging moves to help you regain your strength. Have fun with it, and know that you can make faces, blow kisses, and tickle your baby's tummy or toes. Your baby might even encourage you to do more repetitions of a particular movement, simply because they are giggling or smiling, and take delight in interacting with you.

The exercises shown in this practice are done primarily using a safe grip. As always, please make sure that you are working in a safe environment. I recommend a high-quality sticky yoga mat and urge you to make sure that all toys are out of the way or kept neatly near the front of your mat. Stay responsive to your baby's feedback; it's OK to stop and resume later if you need to feed or change your baby.

Exercise	Page	Focus	Reps/Time
Easy Pose with hand on baby	41	Centering energy	9 slow, deep, centering breaths focusing on the inhalation and the exhalation being equal in length
Unicorn and Rainbow Pose	42	Lower back, abdomen	5 rounds (it's OK to gently tuck the tailbone now that you are postpartum)
Pointer Dog Pose with front hand waving to baby	43	Core stabilization	3-5 deep breaths on the right side, pause in the center to find balance, then 3-5 deep breaths on the left side
Down Dog Pose	44	Lower back, hamstrings, calves	5 slow, steady breaths
Half Sun Salutation with tummy or foot tickles	48	Shoulders, core strength and flexibility	3 rounds; remember that each movement corresponds to an inhalation or exhalation

Exercise	Page	Focus	Reps/Time
Mommy-and-Me Sun Salutation with Kiss-the-Baby Chaturanga	184	Entire body	1-3 rounds of Sun Salutation A; remember that each movement corresponds to an inhalation or exhalation
Squats With Baby	187	Lower body and core	3 sets of 10-12 reps using safe grip (heart to heart or heart to spine)
Shoulder Press With Baby	189	Core stabilizers and shoulders	2 sets of 6-8 reps
Boat Pose With Baby	190	Core with focus on abs, TVA	2 sets of the length of "Row, Row, Row Your Boat"
Flying Baby	191	Core with focus on abs, TVA	2 sets of 8-10 reps
Pigeon Pose while talking to baby	56	Outer thigh, glutes, psoas	9 deep breaths on each side
Easy Twist With Baby	194	Outer thigh and hip	5 deep breaths on the right and then the left
Bridge Pose With Baby	155	Lower back, glutes, hamstrings	5 deep breaths in Bridge Pose while singing "London Bridge"
Deep Relaxation Pose With Baby	66	Entire body	1-3 minutes

OH BABY: FOUNDATIONAL POSTPARTUM PRACTICE

This practice is inspired by your baby's emerging postural muscles and is intended for use when baby is at least four or five months old and has head and neck control. As babies start to gain strength in their back muscles from tummy time, you will notice that they spend a lot of time in yoga postures such as Cobra, Up Dog, and even modified Boat Pose. Their emerging core strength is something they work on all day long, and the movements practiced here are very similar to your baby's movements at four or five months of age. For you, mama, this is past the initial postpartum recovery stage, and the time that you can start to challenge your core stabilizers a little bit more. Note that these are primarily foundational movements to help you rebuild a solid base of strength to support you when lifting your own body weight, so that you can progress to lifting heavier weights if you choose.

Exercise	Page	Focus	Reps/Time
Child's Pose	59	Gently stretches thighs and invites ease	9 slow, deep, centering breaths focusing on the inhalation and the exhalation being equal in length
Hero Pose	195	Warms the abs, TVA, lower back	3 rounds inhaling as you gaze up, exhaling as you round the spine; you can place padding under knees if you wish
Kneeling Sun Salutation With Baby	192	Core stabilization	3-5 deep breaths on the right, pause in the center to find balance, then 3-5 deep breaths on the left
Locust Pose	222	Hamstrings, lower back, arm strength	5 slow deep breaths, feeling heels drawn by gravity toward the earth with each breath
Half Sun Salutation	48	Shoulders, core strength and flexibility	3 rounds; remember that each movement corresponds to an inhalation or exhalation

Exercise	Page	Focus	Reps/Time
Mommy-and-Me Sun Salutation A	184	Shoulders, triceps, core strength and flexibility, hamstrings	3 rounds; remember that each movement corresponds to an inhalation or exhalation
Bridge Into Boat Pose	155, 190	Inner and outer thigh stabilizers, core stabilizers	3-5 deep breaths on the right and then the left
Pigeon Pose	56	Glutes, lower back, hamstrings	9 deep breaths on each side
Supine Hand-to-Big-Toe Pose	167	Outer thighs and hips	5-9 breaths on the right and then the left
Fish Pose	196	Outer thighs, glutes, psoas	9 deep breaths on each side
Deep Relaxation Pose	66	Gently stretches thighs and invites ease	1-3 minutes

Mommy Moves

Six Key Mommy Moves

Over the last ten years, I have tried many different types of traditional exercises and yoga postures with moms and babies. There are six key moves that the Mothers Into Living format incorporates into almost every class. Here are my favorite six moves to enjoy with your baby.

1. *Squats With Baby*: This exercise helps create muscle memory for proper lifting mechanics, in addition to toning and strengthening your lower body.

2. *Lunges With Baby*: This exercise helps strengthen your lower body. This pose can be good to practice with older babies, so that you can rest your baby on your front thigh while supporting the baby's body with your hands around the waist.

3. *Shoulder Press With Baby*: This exercise helps increase the strength of your upper body while baby delights in the movement with mommy.

4. *Flying Baby*: This exercise increases the strength of your core while inviting the spirit of play into your workout with baby.

5. *Bridge Pose With Baby while singing "London Bridge"*: Add song to your Bridge Pose so that as you strengthen your glutes and lower back, your baby begins to learn the words to "London Bridge," accompanied by an up-and-down movement.

6. *Snuggle time*: Taking the time to snuggle and enjoy a little bit of quiet time when neither of you is distracted by external stimuli can be a sweet opportunity to bond.

Information No One Tells You

Diasastis Recti and Mommy-and-Me Workouts

Diasastis recti is a common condition, especially in moms of multiples, moms who are very lean and fit, and deconditioned mamas. Whatever has led to the separation in your abdominal wall, there are exercises to avoid and exercises that can help begin the process of rehabilitation. In extreme cases, surgery might be called for, especially if you've experienced a hernia. The exercise protocol listed in chapter 8 can help begin the process of rehabilitation. It is important to have an assessment by a trained professional such as a physical therapist or an ob/gyn, and in some cases an expert personal trainer, to determine the degree and type of separation.

DR can mean that there is a wide gap between the two sides of the abdominal wall. It can also refer to a deep gap in the connective tissue between the two sides of the rectus abdominis. If you see tenting in your belly when you are rolling out of bed or transitioning from all fours into Down Dog, chances are you have DR. Take the time to get a professional assessment. Remember that the abs work in concert with other core muscles, and when one muscle group has experienced trauma, other muscle groups will often compensate, leading to a muscular imbalance.

It is important to know if you have DR before enjoying the supine mommy-and-me exercises like Flying Baby so that you do not exacerbate an existing problem. Proper carrying mechanics will also be important with DR. You might want to use a front-and-center carrier as opposed to holding baby on your hip for daily activities so that one side of your abdomen does not have to compensate while the other side helps to lift the weight of your baby. If you have any concern or suspicion that you might have DR, I recommend consulting with a physical therapist who specializes in women's health.

Love-Your-Baby Visualization

Gazing Into Each Other's Eyes

There is a form of meditation in which you look into the eyes of your beloved. This form of meditation, called *eye gazing*, is often practiced between couples who are interested in exploring a different or deeper type of connection. The idea is that you explore intimacy by gazing deeply into one another's eyes without looking away. You can enjoy a brief, abbreviated form of this exercise with your baby, and in many cases, feel the soul-to-soul connection when you gaze into your baby's eyes. Follow the suggestions below to try this meditation with your baby.

- Sit comfortably in a rocker or a glider with your baby cradled in your arms.
- Gaze lovingly at your baby and look into your little one's eyes.
- Many times, babies will look deeply into your eyes too. If your baby does not, that is OK; just continue to gaze at their eyes.
- Notice any feelings or thoughts that arise, and try not to judge the experience.
- The whole exercise will last one or two minutes.

Fun Foods

Breastfeeding requires a lot of energy. These yummy energy bites were created by my friend and doula, Lori Bregman. They support the caloric needs of the nursing mama and can potentially increase milk production. Remember that nursing mamas need about 450 to 500 extra calories a day.

Lactation Energy Bites

Contributed by Lori Bregman

> 2 cups rolled oats
>
> 1 cup organic almond butter
>
> 1/2 cup ground flaxseed mixed with 1/2 teaspoon sun chlorella powder
>
> 1 tablespoons brewer's yeast
>
> 1/2 cup organic dark chocolate chips
>
> 1/3 cup honey

Stir ingredients together until mixed well. Chill for 30 minutes until firm, then roll into bite-size balls. Store in the refrigerator or freeze for up to a month for later use. **Yield:** Depends on size of bite-size balls

Belly Blaster Series

In yoga and fitness, the book titles, products, and videos that sell the most are all about the core. I hate to admit it, but I was worried that after I had babies I would never have a flat abdomen again. Even as a fitness professional empowered with the knowledge on how to achieve a flat abdomen, I was concerned that it would not work for me. Trying to get my belly flat before I had babies had always been a challenge, and I was nervous that it would be even harder afterward. Surprisingly, after my second baby, my abdomen is leaner than it has ever been. I've made some basic changes that helped me to work smarter, not harder, and I am happy to share them with you.

Your Body After Baby

My approach to all challenges is to always look to find strength on all levels: physical, mental, and emotional. When looking at why I always held weight in my abdomen, I had to look at the ideas and feelings that I had connected to my belly, in addition to nutrition and exercise. During my first pregnancy, I sent my belly love all day, every day. I realized that I had been so judgmental of this area of my body for so many years that I had created a house for my baby that was full of judgment and negative self-talk. I knew that it was time to send love and light to this area of my body, and to imagine the muscles, tissues, and energetic space filled with positive energy.

I was surprised to find that after the birth of my older son, my belly was flatter than before I was pregnant. I'm not suggesting that sending your belly love is going to make it flat, but I do think that it is important to look at what you might be holding onto in this area. What is your relationship to your belly? Do you look in the mirror and smile? If not, now is a great time to start. Your belly has just performed a miracle; it created a safe space, a sanctuary for your baby to grow and thrive. Take a moment to celebrate the marvelous ability of a woman's body—*your* body—to create space for your little one. If it doesn't feel too out there, you can even thank your belly for a job well done.

Physically, your belly expanded to support your baby. Your ribs and organs gently moved out of the way to create space for your son or daughter. Now that your baby is at least three months old, you can start to explore deeper work in your abdomen. If you are wondering why you need to wait for three months, it's because your body needs time to heal. Many birth professionals refer to this three-month postpartum period as the fourth trimester. The first three months are all about resting, bonding, and settling into your role as a mother.

When you are past the "fourth trimester" and your doctor has cleared you for more intense exercise, you can start deeper core work. The Get Deep practice found in this chapter is intended to help you strengthen the TVA as well as the obliques, lower back, and pelvic floor. These muscles are designed to work in harmony, and while the work is strong and challenging, it is in no way attacking or punishing your belly. Thousands of sit-ups and crunches might give you a line or two in your abs, but this slower, controlled method found in Get Deep is designed to help tone the entire abdomen and lower back, and can give you better definition than crunches alone. It is also designed for functional strength; you're now a mom who needs to lift her baby.

In the practice of yoga, there are many poses and sequences that involve multiple muscle groups working together. An example of this harmony of muscular movement is found in the Sun Salutations, when we warm up the entire body. Bringing your awareness to your core and stabilizing it as you move from Plank through Chaturanga can teach your muscles to work together through functional movements such as bending forward or rising to standing.

I have learned from physical therapists that the deeper muscles of the lower back, the deeper muscles of the abdomen (TVA), the pelvic floor muscles, and the diaphragm all work together in concert. You can feel this when you breathe. Try this simple exercise.

- Sitting in simple cross-legged position, breathe in and notice how your diaphragm and pelvic floor muscles move down.
- Exhale and feel the diaphragm rise (and help to expel the air), and your pelvic floor rises.
- Inhale and feel your diaphragm and pelvic floor move down; exhale and feel them internally lifting.
- Now shift your attention to your abdomen and inhale. Notice how your belly expands as you inhale.
- Exhale and feel your abdomen gently move in toward the midline, like a corset.
- Continue to breathe in and feel the belly expand, and breathe out and feel it gently contract.
- Now put all of this together: Inhale to feel your diaphragm moving down, your pelvic floor moving down, and your abdomen expanding.
- Exhale and feel your diaphragm moving up, your pelvic floor moving up, and your abdomen contracting.

Noticing how our muscles work together as we breathe is very similar to the yogic principle of bandhas. In Sanskrit, the word *bandha* means lock. There are four main bandhas, or locks, that can be engaged in the body.

1. *Mula bandha, or Root Lock*: *Mula* means *root*; its Sanskrit name is similar to that of the root chakra, because mula bandha occurs at the level of the root chakra. It is the upward-lifting energy of the pelvic floor.

2. *Uddiyanabandha, or Belly Lock*: *Uddiyana* means *to fly in and up*; it refers to an energetic lift at the level of the abdomen. The external or physical expression is the contraction of the TVA and the rectus abdominis.

3. *Jalandarabandha, or Throat Lock*: Not commonly practiced in the West, the throat lock involves a form of breath control that allows you to extend the length of the breath. The external expression involves tucking the chin in toward the neck.

4. *Mahabandha, or Supreme Lock*: This lock engages all three of these locks simultaneously.

You can see how the body's locks, or bandhas, are similar to what Paul Chek, a renowned exercise physiologist, calls the *inner unit*. This phrase refers to the diaphragm at the top, the pelvic floor at the bottom, the TVA in the front, and the multifidi in the back. You can envision this as an inner cylinder of power that works together to help your body perform whatever task is needed. The ancient yogic explanation is quite similar, with strength and awareness held at the same three levels of the body. Looking at the similarities of the Eastern and Western teachings shows us that the different parts of the body work together like musicians working together in a symphony: Each part has its assigned role and all work together to create something magnificent. In this particular example, something magnificent might be the simple act of lifting your baby up for a kiss while engaging your pelvic floor (so there is no LBL), your abs (so there is no lower back pain), and gently tucking your chin while kissing your baby.

Exercise After Baby

In 25 years of fitness and yoga, I have seen many different abdominal machines, devices, and moves that range from very effective to very silly. Years ago I was taught that it was important to create a program that included a move for each part of the abdomen: lower abs, upper abs, and obliques. But information changes and evolves, so it's important to stay current with education. I spent years doing crunches, ab rolling, ab slinging, and side bending. What I learned is that while these moves can give you a bit of definition, real strength and those deeper abdominal cuts come with a different type of training. Total body moves and sequences are surprisingly effective and can set you up for success in reclaiming your core strength after giving birth.

While it would seem logical to zero in on specific parts of the body, we actually burn more calories and teach the body to work as a functional unit when we enjoy total body movements. Crunches, which are a staple for many trainers in program design, can help strengthen the abs but they only

The Three Main Body Types

In fitness, we often speak of three main body types, or somatotypes. Each of these three types, ectomorph, mesomorph, and endomorph, has a distinctive build (see figure 10.1).

- *Ectomorphs* tend to be leaner with less body fat than the other two body types.
- *Mesomorphs* tend to be more muscular and put on muscle mass more easily than the other two body types.
- *Endomorphs* are more pear-shaped and carry more fat in the lower body.

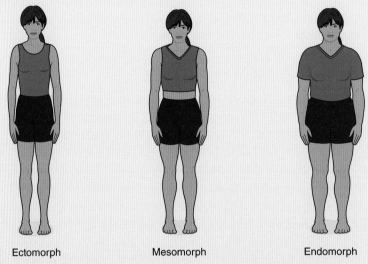

Ectomorph   Mesomorph   Endomorph

Figure 10.1 The three main body types: ectomorph, mesomorph, and endomorph.

In Ayurvedic medicine, there is a similar system of categorizing body types, with slightly more emphasis on noting which maladies or diseases tend to be present in each of the three. Ayurvedic practitioners recommend specific ways of eating depending on your *dosha* or body type, and balancing your type for optimum health. The following explains a little bit about each *dosha*, and which foods are said to help achieve balance.

- *Kappha (Earth):* Typically bigger build, slower digestion, slower metabolism, tendency toward seasonal allergies. Emphasize pungent foods like onions and garlic. Avoid refined sugar, such as candy and desserts.
- *Pitta (Fire):* Warm-bodied, intense, goal oriented, prone to having rashes, inflammation, and heartburn. Emphasize cool and bitter foods, such as kale salad. Avoid pungent, spicy food such as hot chilies.
- *Vatta (Air):* The leanest of all of the builds. Energetic and creative, tendency toward brain fog and worrying too much, tendency toward constipation. Emphasize sweet foods that are warm and grounding in nature, such as sweet potato soup. Avoid cold carbonated drinks.

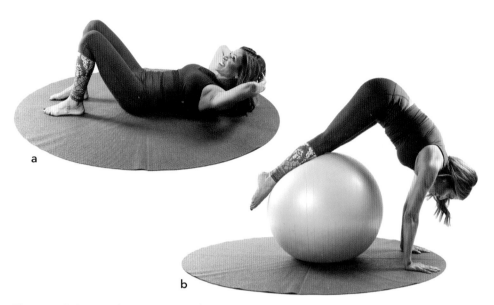

Figure 10.2 Working one muscle groups as in a crunch (a) versus multiple muscle groups, as in a Pike on a stability ball (b).

target the upper part of the abs (see figure 10.2a). For that reason, it is far more efficient to do a total body movement like a Pike on a stability ball (see figure 10.2b). Piking on the ball will work the stabilizers of your shoulders and your core. This simply means that while you are focusing primarily on the front of your belly and your lower back in this exercise, your obliques and the muscles that support your scapula are active too. For busy moms, it can be far more efficient to enjoy total body movement to get stronger and more defined. This type of training not only saves time but also feels more playful and less like a chore.

Nutrition for the Body and Belly

It is important to remember that it is not just how we train the abdomen that makes it look and feel strong from the inside out. Proper nutrition is the key to getting the results that you desire. There are varying opinions in the fitness community about how your food impacts the way you look. Most trainers will tell you that at least 50 percent of what you eat determines how you look, with some trainers going so far as to say it is closer to 70 percent. Either way, it is clear that the old trainer adage, "Abs are cooked in the kitchen," is alive and well.

Making sure that you have the proper fuel in your system will give you energy, and making sure that you eat foods that agree with your digestive system will help you avoid bloating and discomfort. With all of the conflicting advice, it can be challenging to know which way of eating is best for you: paleo, vegan, ketogenic, raw. There are hundreds of ways of eating and no one way will work for everyone. Here are some basic guidelines that can help to set you up for success.

- Drink water; our bodies need water, and water has been shown to increase energy.
- Choose real, natural foods that will give you more energy than over-processed foods.
- Eat fruits and vegetables every day, as they contain vital minerals and vitamins.
- Don't eat anything you wouldn't feed your baby; if it's not good for baby, is it something you want to put into your own body?
- Eat the rainbow; a colorful variety of many different foods will help you get the full range of nutrients your body needs.

Ayurvedic medicine encourages people to follow most of these nutrition guidelines. There is a large emphasis on eating the rainbow and making sure that you enjoy different tastes (sweet, sour, salty, and so on). Many yogis choose their food based on the Ayurvedic principles discussed in the Three Main Body Types sidebar earlier in this chapter. One tip that you might not see in the Ayurvedic texts that I have added to this list is to eat what you feed your baby. This tip comes from my personal experience as a mom and as a trainer. One day while giving my son water to drink, he asked me for a sip of my double espresso. I realized at that moment that I wanted to be an example of health and wellness for him, and if I wouldn't give it to him, why was I choosing it for myself? I share this advice with moms and dads all the time as it is a great test of whether what you are about to eat is truly healthy.

While we all crave a little energy lift or a sweet treat now and then, we can set ourselves up for success by choosing foods that we would be happy to provide for our children. Generally speaking we eat breakfast, lunch, and dinner seven days a week, with some snacks here and there. That means that we have at least 21 chances to get it right. If you have 20 clean meals and choose one less healthy meal a week, you set yourself up for being able to achieve your goals. The overall pattern is healthy, and an occasional cheat meal is OK. Many bodybuilders and fitness professionals purposely build in a cheat meal to their weekly calendar. The cheat meal can give you a psychological boost and helps you to avoid feeling deprived. Some nutritionists even say that the cheat meal can help you to move past a weight loss plateau by raising your metabolic rate.

Stabilizing Blood Sugar

In the 1990s, biochemist Barry Sears wrote a famous book, *Zone Diet*; it was the first book in mainstream publications to speak about stabilizing blood sugar. The basic concept behind the book is that we need a specific ratio of fat, carbohydrate, and protein. The ratio proposed in the text is 30-40-30, with 30 percent fat, 40 percent carbohydrate, and 30 percent protein. Finding a one-size-fits-all diet is nearly impossible, but this particular book raised our awareness that certain foods can spike your blood sugar, which can lead to a subsequent drop, or energy crash. By balancing our meals, we help stabilize our blood sugar.

Foods that are high in refined sugar will spike your blood sugar. We all know that candy and many desserts contain a lot of sugar, but what can be surprising is how many other foods also have high amounts of sugar. Pasta, bread, tortillas, cereal, and soda can all spike the level of blood sugar in your body. If you are categorized as prediabetic, the constant elevation of glucose (blood sugar) can lead to insulin resistance and diabetes. Many websites and books have long lists of the glycemic index for each food. These lists can tell you which foods will tend to spike your glucose levels.

Finding a balance of carbohydrate, protein, and fat in each meal can help to stabilize your blood sugar levels. Each individual's ideal ratio might be slightly different from the next person's. Also, depending on what phase of motherhood you are in, you have different nutritional needs. For example, if you are breastfeeding, you will need a slight increase in your caloric intake. Having another serving of vegetables or fruit can increase the calories in a healthy way, and taking the time to add a little almond butter on top of an apple or a little bit of lowfat cheese on your broccoli will add fat and protein to your extra serving of carbs (fruit and veggies).

Some moms do really well with eating every three hours to maintain blood sugar levels, while others swear by occasional fasting or juicing. *Your Strong, Sexy Pregnancy* is all about what makes you feel strong and sexy from the inside out. Take time to experiment with different food combinations and allow the experience to be enjoyable. You can invite the feeling of adventure and play into everything you do, including eating.

Identifying How Foods Make You Feel

Whichever way of eating resonates with you because of culture, religion, taste, or budget, you can start to take note of which foods leave you feeling great an hour later, and which foods leave you feeling lethargic, bloated, or gassy. Digestion is an important topic in nutrition, and I encourage you to play with different food combinations, and even keep a photographic food journal. For most moms, the thought of taking the time to write down serving sizes of everything they eat and drink is not realistic, especially if they also need to keep track of the time they ate. However, chances are that you have a smartphone or tablet with a lot of memory on it (for the thousands of pictures of adorable kids), so you can take a photo of whatever you eat. At the end of the day, scroll through your photos and notice the quantities of food and the time stamp on the pictures.

Also notice how you felt throughout the day. Were you energetic and feeling great? Did you get *hangry* (so hungry that you were angry)? If you felt tired, irritable, or hangry, chances are you did not eat the correct ratio of fats, proteins, and carbs for your body. Rather than dictate your best way of eating, my best advice is for you to become a detective and look at what is best for your body. What makes you feel strong, energetic, and a happy mom?

Which Way of Eating Is Best?

There are many different ways of eating, and it's up to every woman to decide what works best for her. Here is a basic guide to a few different styles of creating a healthy diet.

- *Vegan*: Does not eat eggs, dairy products, or any other product derived from an animal.
- *Vegetarian*: Does not eat any animal flesh, whether meat, fish, or fowl.
- *Pescatarian*: Same as a vegetarian, but with the addition of fish.
- *Lacto/ovo vegetarian*: Does not eat animal flesh, but will eat eggs and dairy products.
- *Paleo*: Eats vegetables, fruits, nuts, roots, and meats. Avoids processed foods. Based on the paleo diet, which reflects early man's ability to hunt and gather.
- *Ketogenic*: High in protein and fat, low in carbohydrate. Forces the body to burn more fat.
- *Macrobiotic*: Said to balance yin and yang (masculine and feminine energies); emphasizes locally grown whole-grain cereals, legumes, vegetables, seaweed, fermented soy products, and fruit.

Please note that food is not entertainment. If you read that last sentence and maybe thought *Pizza makes me happy*, I totally get it. We all have a cheat food that we enjoy occasionally. But try to think of food as fuel; if we put low-grade fuel (donuts, fast food, sugary soda) in our bodies, we usually feel uncomfortable. The discomfort might be gas, bloating, energy crash, skin breakouts, and so on. Instead, fuel your body with high-quality foods that you know will keep you feeling great and comfortable. Being doubled over in pain from gas and indigestion makes it really hard to feel strong or sexy, and in my opinion, you deserve to feel great. You are the heart of the family and my goal is to help you look and feel fantastic.

Yoga Poses and Exercises After Baby

Throughout your pregnancy, your core muscles created a safe home for your baby. Now that it is time to reclaim this space and your strength, take your time as you reignite the fire in your belly. It is important not to attack the abs. Instead, focus on rebuilding strength from the inside out. It can be helpful to envision your abdominal muscles as a corset and feel the corset helping you to gently draw in at the end of each exhalation. Your yoga practice will naturally call on the strength of your core muscles as stabilizers. Take your time rebuilding this strong foundation, and do not be surprised if you find that by patiently building the "powerhouse muscles," you can be even stronger than you were before pregnancy.

Forearm Side Plank Pose

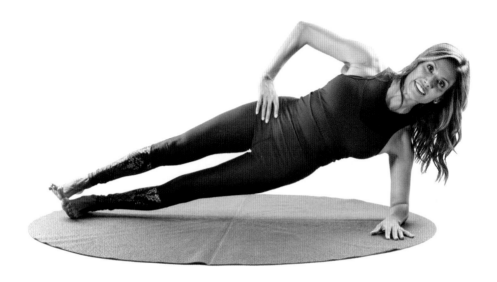

Benefits

This pose strengthens the obliques and core stabilizers.

Feeling

Feel the strength in the side of your abdomen as you hover above the floor. You might remember when planking was a trend. Around that same time, there were also a lot of folks who were able to hold their bodies parallel with the ground while holding onto a street sign, like a human flag. All of these exercises use your body weight to hover above the ground, and give deep knowledge and awareness of how to use the weight. Yogis call this uddiyana bandha, or belly lock; the awareness of holding the deeper abdominal muscles in a contraction is what allows these types of longer holds. Explore your strength as you start to learn about biomechanics from the inside out, and don't forget to invite a sense of play.

Instruction

- Begin lying down on the floor on your left side.
- Place your left forearm on the floor and lift your hips off the floor (see figure). Your left hand can rest on your left hip.
- Feel your right hip stacked on top of your left hip as you engage the strength of your entire core, focusing on the obliques.
- Hold for 30 to 60 seconds, and then change sides.

Adjustments

To make this exercise more challenging, you can lift the top leg so that it hovers about four to six inches above the bottom leg. Make sure that you continue to keep your hips and shoulders stacked.

Pike Pose on Stability Ball

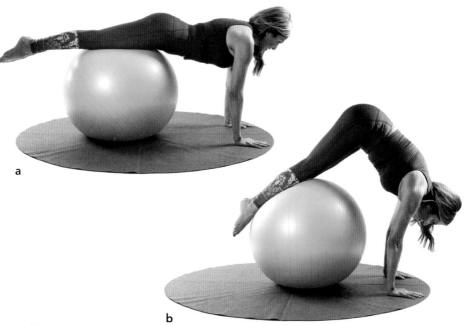

a

b

Benefits

This exercise strengthens the core stabilizers with emphasis on the TVA and the abs.

Feeling

If you've ever watched the Summer Olympics, you've probably seen divers come into Pike position and sometimes even touch their toes. Channel your inner athlete and use your strength to make the ball glide in a steady motion. It is often the most challenging exercises that look the easiest from the outside. Be patient with yourself as you find your balance and work toward a graceful and fluid motion in this exercise.

Instruction

▌ Begin with your abdomen lying on the stability ball and your hands on the floor.
▌ Slowly walk your hands forward and allow the ball to roll down the length of the front of your legs (see figure a) until the tops of your feet (or your shoelaces if you are wearing athletic shoes) are on the ball, and your hands are directly underneath your shoulders in push-up (Plank) position.
▌ Exhale and use your abdominal strength to contract your abs as you lift your hips into Pike position (see figure b).
▌ Inhale to return to the starting position. Repeat.

Adjustments

If for any reason there is a challenge with balance or if you do not have a stability ball, you can turn the exercise upside down into Boat Pose, which is also a Pike position. If you choose Boat Pose, you can let the upper and lower body lower slowly on the inhalation and then exhale as you lift into Boat Pose or Pike.

Prone Leg Lift on Stability Ball

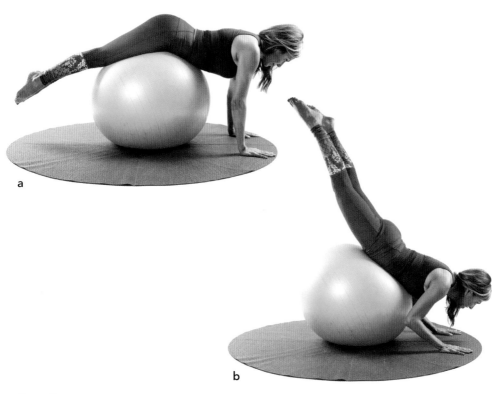

a

b

Benefits

This exercise strengthens the core stabilizers with emphasis on the lower back and the hamstrings.

Feeling

This exercise is fun and can be approached with a lighthearted attitude. Try to envision your legs as a dolphin's tail splashing in and out of the water.

Instruction

- Begin with your abdomen lying on the stability ball and your hands on the floor (see figure a). Your hands should be shoulder width apart and the shoulders aligned with your wrists.
- Keep your feet a few inches wider than hip width as you exhale and lift your legs high into the air (see figure b).
- Inhale as you slowly lower your legs and straighten your arms.
- Exhale; your elbows will naturally bend a little as you lift your legs and feel the strength in your lower back and hamstrings.

Adjustments

Beginners can lift one leg at a time. Alternate the leg lift until you feel confident in lifting both legs together.

Supine Stability Ball Pass

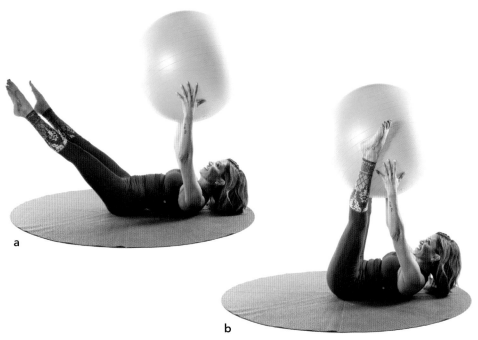

a

b

Benefits

This exercise strengthens the core stabilizers with emphasis on the abs, TVA, and psoas.

Feeling

Most exercises with the stability ball are playful in nature; it feels as though you're working with a giant beach ball, especially if you choose the variation and play catch with your feet. Remember that fitness can be fun!

Instruction

- Begin lying on your back with your arms extended overhead and a stability ball between your hands (see figure a).
- Slowly lift your upper body and legs into Inverted Pike Pose (Boat Pose), and pass the ball from your hands to your feet (see figure b).
- Allow your upper and lower body to droop until your legs, arms, head, and shoulders hover above the floor.
- Rise back up into Inverted Pike and pass the ball from your feet to your hands. Repeat several times.

Adjustments

To make the exercise more challenging, you can throw the ball toward your legs and catch the ball between your ankles. In this variation, you still pass the ball from your feet to your hands while you are in the crunch position but you throw the ball every time it is in your hands.

Seated Twist

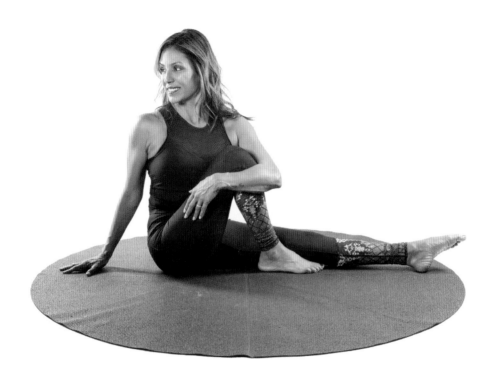

Benefits

This pose works the core stabilizers with an emphasis on the obliques.

Feeling

Twists are detoxifying in nature. Yoga teachers like to say that when you are doing twists you are wringing out what your body no longer needs.

Instruction

- Begin seated on the floor with your legs extended straight in front of you. Bend your right knee and place your right foot flat on the floor.
- Place your right hand on the floor, about 10-12 inches behind your hip.
- Inhale and lift your left arm to the sky as you feel your spine lengthening.
- Exhale and twist the upper body to the right. Bring your left arm to the outside of the right knee, and turn the right palm away from your body (see figure).
- Continue to breathe deeply, and remember that the exhalation is the entrance to a deeper pose. This simply means that every time you exhale, you release the air, which lets you twist a little bit deeper, if that is comfortable for your body.
- After several breath cycles, pause, and change sides.

Adjustments

You may place a folded blanket underneath your sit bones for comfort.

Sufi Roll

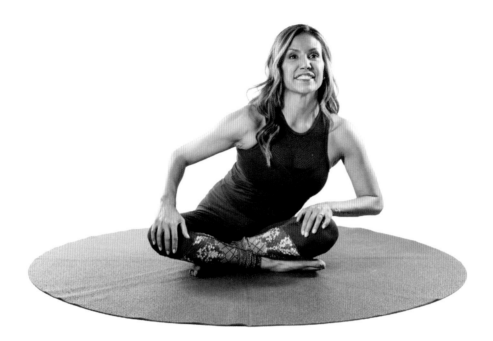

Benefits

This exercise gently warms the muscles of the core stabilizers.

Feeling

Connect to the feeling of your sit bones pressing gently into the earth, and the strong, stable foundation that your lower body provides. Allow your upper body to move freely. In the esoteric teachings of yoga, the lower body corresponds to the element of earth, and the spine corresponds to the element of water. Feel the sense of grounding in the lower body and fluidity in the upper body.

Instruction

- Begin seated on the floor with your legs crossed in Easy Pose. Feel your sit bones on the floor.
- Allow your upper body to move gently to the left in a circular motion (see figure). Note that this very gentle movement is also safe during pregnancy.
- After several circles of the upper body in one direction, pause to find center, and then change sides.

Adjustments

You can place a folded blanket underneath your sit bones for comfort.

Pilates Roll-Down

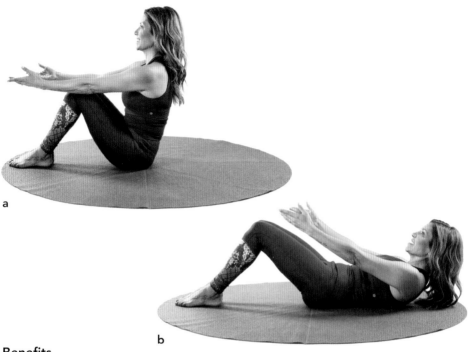

a

b

Benefits

This exercise works the core stabilizers, with emphasis on the abdomen and lower back.

Feeling

There is a feeling of rising in the upper body and reaching your hands up, as though to reach for the hands of another person. Think of trapeze artists lifting their hands so that another person can grab hold of them. Imagine that someone is standing above you to help lift you. In reality, it will be your breath as well as your deep internal core strength that help to lift you.

Instruction

▌ Begin in a seated position on the floor with your knees bent and your feet pressing into the floor (see figure a). Reach your arms straight ahead.

▌ Inhale and lower your body toward the mat, making sure to keep the spine long, and the breastbone lifted as you lower (see figure b).

▌ Exhale and rise back up to the starting position.

Adjustments

It is challenging to keep your feet flat on the floor when you first learn this exercise. You can slide your toes under the bottom edge of your sofa to help you keep your feet on the floor. If you choose this option, make sure to keep your knees bent. If you have a toddler or a young child, you can ask them to sit on your feet and make it a game to help mommy get stronger like a superhero.

Pilates Roll-Down With Oblique Twist

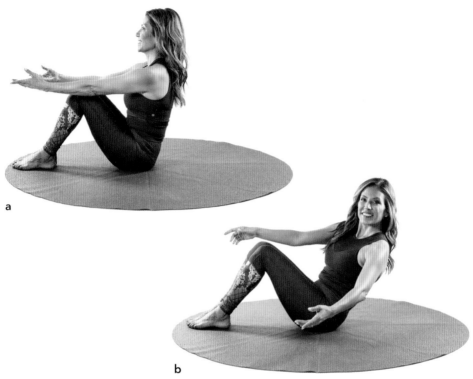

a

b

Benefits

This exercise works the core stabilizers, with emphasis on the waist.

Feeling

Olympic ice skaters have decades of training experience that makes their movements look easy. Making a challenging movement look graceful takes a tremendous amount of strength. Do this movement with ease and grace so that it looks as though you're gliding from side to side. Move slowly and channel your inner Olympian.

Instruction

- Begin seated on the floor with your knees bent and your feet pressing into the floor (see figure a).
- Inhale and reach your arms out to the sides and twist your torso to the left as you begin to lower your upper body to a 45 degree angle (see figure b).
- Rise back up to the starting position with the upper body facing straight ahead, and repeat on the right with the upper body twisting to the right as you lower.
- Alternate sides and return to center after each repetition. Make sure that each time you twist, it is a slow, controlled motion, and that your lower back is protected by moving smoothly between movements.

Adjustments

As with the preceding exercise, you can place your feet under the edge of your sofa, or ask your small child to sit on your feet.

Pointer Dog Pose With Abdominal Flexion

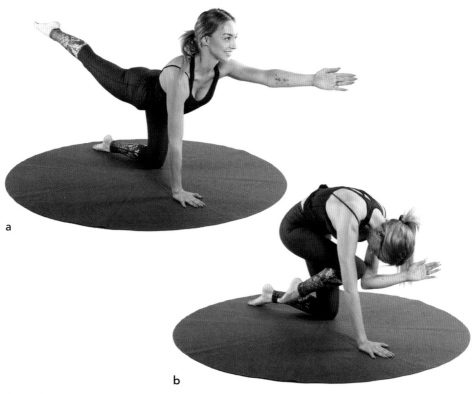

a

b

Benefits

This movement strengthens the TVA and the abs.

Feeling

Yogis and many other Eastern practitioners correlate the abdominal area to the element of fire. Imagine that every time you draw your knee in, you are stoking the flames of strength in your belly.

Instruction

- Begin on all fours with your feet hip width apart and your hands shoulder width apart.
- Reach the left arm forward and your right leg back while inhaling (see figure a).
- Exhale and draw the elbow to the knee while rounding the spine (see figure b). Focus on the strength in your deep abdominal muscles each time you draw the elbow to the knee, and exhale.
- Repeat the movement for the desired number of repetitions, then repeat on the other side.

Adjustments

You can place a folded blanket under your knees for extra padding.

Locust Pose

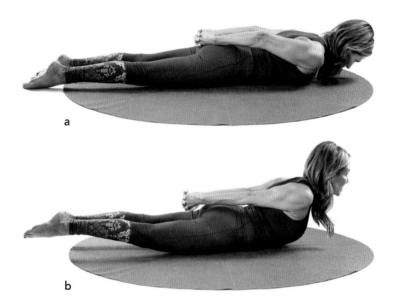

a

b

Benefits

This pose strengthens the core stabilizers, with emphasis on the lower back.

Feeling

In fitness, this exercise is traditionally called superman. In yoga, it's referred to as Locust Pose. Whichever you call it, it gives you a feeling of flying. Let your body feel very light in the air as you focus on the strength of your lower back helping you lift with power and grace.

Instruction

- Begin lying on your abdomen with your legs straight and your extended arms resting on your glutes with your fingers interlaced. Your feet should be hip width apart (see figure a).
- Slowly lift your legs, chest, and head off the yoga mat and your arms off of your glutes, drawing your ankles together (see figure b). You will feel a strong muscular contraction in your lower back.
- Control the descent as you slowly lower your entire body back to the floor. Repeat.

Adjustment

The intensity of this exercise depends on simple physics: The longer the lever, the more work is required. To make this exercise a little bit easier, keep your arms back at your sides. The lower back will still be active, but this is a great option if you are working with shoulder injury or sensitivity. You can also place a folded blanket under your hip bones for extra comfort.

Sphinx Pose

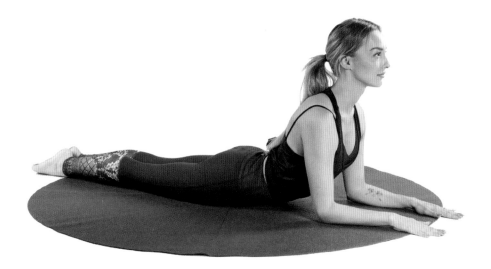

Benefits

This pose strengthens the lower back while stretching the abdomen.

Feeling

Like the Egyptian Sphinx, find a sense of calm and noble strength in this pose by breathing deeply and allowing your heart to rise. Lift the crown of your head to the sky in this regal pose and feel your graceful neck elongate.

Instruction

- Lie down on the floor on your abdomen with your legs straight behind you, hip width apart. Rotate the legs slightly inward.
- Place your forearms on your yoga mat as you lift your upper body. Gently draw your shoulder blades in toward your spine (this is called scapular retraction).
- Lengthen your spine and lift your chest as you breathe deeply into this gentle backbend (see figure).

Adjustments

You can place a folded blanket under your hip bones for additional cushioning.

Putting It All Together

Once you have established a baseline of strength, flexibility, and cardio-vascular endurance from the Mommy-and-Me practices in the preceding chapter, it's time to up the ante a little bit. With your doctor's clearance, you can add the postnatal core practices at the end of this chapter to help challenge your core strength. These practices specifically target the deeper abdominal muscles and can assist with proper posture as well as with regaining a flatter belly.

Mommy Move

Belly Fat Blasters

When targeting your abdomen, it's important to train the upper abdominal muscles, the lower abdominal muscles, and the obliques. The Deep Core exercise program includes exercises for all three. When you feel you have mastered these movements, you can graduate to a more advanced movement that will blast belly fat. Think back to high school gym class; I'm sure you'll remember Burpees!

Burpees are fast and effective, and they train your body as a whole. For many of my private clients, this straightforward exercise can make the difference between a core that just feels strong and a core that also *looks* strong. I believe that function is more important than form, but I know that we all like to look great too. If you are going to work hard, seeing the results can give you extra motivation to continue on your health and fitness path. See chapter 11 for instructions on how to do a Burpee.

Information No One Tells You

Using a Postpartum Belt

Many companies make corsetlike belts for moms to wear after giving birth. These belts or bindings are common in many cultures. In Mexico, many women use such a belt, called a *faja*, after labor and delivery. In the United States, these products are often endorsed by a celebrity and have ornate stitching or lace designs to make them look more like lingerie. The purpose of these compression garments is to help support the abdominal muscles and lower back while the uterus undergoes the process of involution (contracting back to its normal size). More and more women are starting to use these belts beyond the first 40 days postpartum. Here are a few pros and cons for your consideration.

Pros

- They provide support for the core.
- They're great for those who have DR or hernia.
- They apply compression.

Cons

- They can be uncomfortable or itchy.
- They are expensive, especially if you need a high-end belt with extra comfort for C-section incision.
- Core muscles sometime become dependent on the external support.
- If the belt is too tight, LBL can occur when you squat, because of the additional pressure.

Love-Your-Baby Visualization

Love Your Post-Baby Body

I like to offer this visualization to moms who are nursing or bottle-feeding, because it is a sweet meditation you can do while feeding or cradling your baby. Begin sitting up tall in your glider or on your sofa. Cradling your beautiful baby, close your eyes and slow your breath down. Feel the softness of the front of your body, specifically your breasts and your abdomen. Notice how comfortably your baby snuggles into the front of your body. Bring your attention to your belly and notice if you are holding judgment around this part of your body. What are the first three words that come up for you when you tap into how you think of your belly? If any of these words is judgmental or harsh, simply notice and try to let go of criticism as you connect to your baby snuggling against this softer part of your body. This soft part was your baby's home for approximately 40 weeks and created a safe space for your child to grow. Take a moment to thank your belly for its miraculous ability to house, nourish, and protect your baby.

Now take a moment to think about how you would like your abdomen to feel. Would you like your core to feel strong, supported, and powerful? Notice the words that come up as you reflect on what you wish to call in and create. Breathe into the feeling of strength as you sit up a little bit taller, like a queen. Thank your body for the ability to transform, to adapt to the different stages of your life. Let your body know your intention. For example, if your intention is to strengthen your core, feel your inner corset muscles gently weaving together and let your body and your mind know that you are now moving from carrying a baby inside you to carrying a baby in your arms. Set your intention so that your future workouts are inspired by your vision. Slowly flutter your eyes open and know that, by setting a clear intention, you have begun the process of reclaiming your core strength.

Fun Foods

While training at Gold's Gym in Venice Beach, California, I had the pleasure of meeting athlete and entrepreneur Shannan Yorton Penna. The creator of Quest bars, Shannan is a genius at creating balanced, healthy choices that taste amazing. Here is her recipe for yummy cheesecakes.

Personal Crustless Cheesecakes
Contributed by Shannan Yorton Penna, Quest Creator

> 4 eggs
>
> 8 ounces sour cream
>
> 8 ounces cream cheese
>
> 3 to 4 tablespoons lemon juice
>
> 1 tablespoon lemon zest
>
> 1/8 teaspoon pure powdered sucralose, or about 1/2 cup erythritol
>
> 1 teaspoon vanilla bean seeds
>
> 1 cup blanched almond flour
>
> 1 scoop Quest protein powder (vanilla or unflavored)

Preheat oven to 350°. Combine ingredients in a large bowl. Spoon batter into muffin tins. Bake for 35 to 40 minutes, or until cheesecakes are not wet in the middle and the tops are dry to the touch.

Yield: Makes 4-8 mini cheesecakes depending on tin size.

GET DEEP: POSTNATAL CORE CHALLENGE PRACTICE

Recovering strength in the deep abdominal muscles takes patience. Once you have laid a strong foundation with the postpartum exercises in chapters 8 and 9, you can start to explore more intense and challenging movements, intended for moms who are at least four months postpartum. Take your time with these exercises; slow, deliberate, safe movement can increase your strength more effectively than ballistic (fast or bouncy) movement. As always, listen to your body and rest when you need to, while remembering that the mind often gives up before the body. Stay strong, mama; you've got this! Note that a stability ball is needed for this practice.

Exercise	Page	Focus	Reps/Time
Mountain Pose	45	Centering energy	5 slow, deep, centering breaths, focusing on the inhalation and the exhalation being equal in length
Half Sun Salutation	48	Shoulders, core strength and flexibility	3 rounds; remember that each movement corresponds to an inhalation or exhalation
Sun Salutation A	52	Shoulders, triceps, core strength and flexibility, hamstrings	3 rounds; remember that each movement corresponds to an inhalation or exhalation
Forearm Plank Pose	161	TVA, abs, lower back, obliques	30-second holds; 2 sets
Forearm Side Plank Pose	213	Obliques, triceps	3-5 deep breaths with the right elbow on the floor, then 3-5 deep breaths with the left elbow on the floor; option to repeat on both sides
Pike Pose on Stability Ball	214	TVA, abs, lower back, obliques	3 sets of 8-10 reps

Exercise	Page	Focus	Reps/Time
Prone Leg Lift on Stability Ball	215	Lower back and hamstrings	3 sets of 10-12 reps
Supine Stability Ball Pass	216	Core stabilizers	3 sets of 10-12 reps
Seated Twist	217	Stretching the core stabilizers	5 deep breaths right and left
Seated meditation in Easy Pose	41	Calming the entire body and mind	2-5 minutes or until you feel a sense of completion

CORE SET: POSTNATAL CORE RECOVERY PRACTICE

Remember that the core muscles act like a corset; they help keep everything drawn in toward the midline so you can stand tall like a queen. This practice is intended for those who are at least three to four months postpartum. Take your time with this workout, as it is meant to be practiced at a slow, steady pace. Try using music that parallels your heartbeat. An example of a song that has about 95 beats per minute is "No Woman, No Cry" by Bob Marley. Note that you need a thicker yoga or Pilates mat for comfort on the floor for this practice.

Exercise	Page	Focus	Reps/Time
Sufi Roll	218	Warms up the core	15 to the right, deep breath, 15 to the left, deep breath
Unicorn and Rainbow Pose	42	Warms the abs, TVA, lower back	3 rounds inhaling as you gaze up, exhaling as you round the spine; 3 more rounds adding lion's breath as the exhale
Pointer Dog Pose With Abdominal Flexion	221	Abs as flexors and obliques as stabilizers	5 reps with right arm forward and left leg back; 5 reps with left arm forward and right leg back
Bridge Into Boat Pose	155, 190	Lower back, TVA, abs	10 reps of each pose, at a slow, gliding pace
Pilates Roll-Down	219	Lower back, TVA, abs	2 sets of 8-10 reps
Pilates Roll-Down with Oblique Twist	220	Lower back, TVA, abs, obliques	2 sets of 8-10 reps
Locust Pose	222	Lower back	2 sets of 8-10 reps
Sphinx Pose	223	Abdomen	5-10 slow, deep breaths
Child's Pose	59	Lower back, obliques	15 slow, deep breaths

Self-Care for Moms

When I was pregnant I felt I had control over what was happening with my sons. As soon as they were born, I realized that control was an illusion, and that all children have their own paths. There will be some days when kids can't sleep, are teething, or refuse to eat what you made for lunch. Surrendering the illusion of control can be a powerful lesson. What we learn in the practice of yoga is that the only thing we really have control of in life is how we react to any given situation. I have found that good self-care can empower you with patience for choosing your actions and reactions to the joys and challenges of being a mom.

Self-care in the form of good sleep, healthy foods, and exercise can sometimes feel indulgent when we have little ones to take care of. As moms, we sometimes get caught in what I call *mom guilt*. I've heard moms say that they do not, or cannot, work out because they put their kids first. I don't subscribe to this way of thinking. Of course my children come first, but the choice is not between my health and my children. My dear friend and doula Lori Bregman taught me to apply the airplane principle to motherhood. If there is trouble on a plane, the parents need to put on their own oxygen mask first, so they can then effectively help the child. Of course I'm not comparing ab workouts to the seriousness of airplane trouble, but it's important to remember that we have to take good care of ourselves so that we can take good care of our children. Running on no sleep, eating our children's leftover food, and not having a good routine for self-care is a recipe for a depleted mama. Taking care of your body, mind, and spirit will not only allow you to support your children, it will also model good self-care for them.

Get Enough Sleep

Sleep is an often-overlooked part of fitness. Doctors say that on average, we should get eight hours of sleep each night. If you are a new mom, I know that might not be possible with nighttime feedings and needing to check on your little one, so it becomes that much more important that the sleep that you get is quality sleep.

Proper sleep can help with all of the systems of your body, including the endocrine system, which helps to regulate the body's hormones. Insulin is a hormone that allows your body to use the sugar from carbohydrates as energy. Lack of sleep has been linked to insulin resistance. Chronic sleep loss is likely to promote the development of insulin resistance, a risk factor for obesity and diabetes. And, research shows that those with sufficient sleep, burn more fat than their under-rested counterparts. Also, lack of rest makes you crave food, especially sugar, and can slow down your body's ability to break down sugar. To help offset how inadequate sleep affects the body, here are some simple ways to help you sleep better.

- Exercise regularly.
- Leave your electronics outside of the bedroom, as the blue light can disturb your sleep.
- Try to stick with a regular sleep schedule as much as possible.
- Create a sleep ritual, similar to the way that we create bedtime rituals for babies.
- Put a few drops of lavender oil on your pillow at night.
- Keep your room cool and comfortable.
- Listen to a guided meditation before bed.
- Avoid heavy meals before bedtime.

When I was growing up, there was a commercial showing a mom who looked like a hot mess in a pink robe, saying "Calgon, take me away." Magically, she was whisked into a bubble bath with a peaceful, well-rested look on her face. We've all had days like this, when we want to be rescued from the grind of daily life. As a new mom, you'll have days when you feel sleep deprived, with spit-up on your shoulder, and wonder when there will be time to take a shower. On those days when you feel like you dream about a warm bubble bath and a nap, but don't have the time, an ancient yoga technique might just do the trick.

Yoga nidra means yogic sleep, and the practice can leave you feeling refreshed and renewed. Dr. Kamini Desai, director of the Amrit Yoga Institute, describes yoga nidra as "Emptying progressively the contents of the mind by moving down through progressive brain wave states, where there are naturally less and less thoughts." As a mom it is completely normal for you to have a long running to-do list ever present in your mind. Yoga nidra can help your mind slow down and let go of the constant I should do thoughts, and rest your body and your mind.

Allowing the mind and the body to rest is an integral part of health and wellness, but an often forgotten one. I know that as a busy mom, you probably don't always get all the sleep you need. Yoga nidra is an easy way to find a quick respite. Here is a lovely guided yoga nidra practice, as contributed by a wonderful yoga teacher, master of traditional oriental Medicine, and mom, Kali Alexander.

- Take a moment to get settled. Lie down on your back with pillows beneath your knees and your head. Gently rock side to side a few times, allowing your body to find comfort. Take a few cycles of a slow deep breath through your nose, hold it for a couple of seconds, then sigh it out through your mouth. Now let your body spread out like Sunday morning pancake batter.

- Close your eyes and rest the heels of your hands over your eyelids.

- Allow your feet to drop away from the midline. Feel your legs relax, your hips become heavy, and your belly soften. Soften through the center of your chest and allow the weight of your head to surrender to gravity.

- Call forth an intention. Simply refine your intention to a single word. If many words come to mind, know that the one intention you choose is the gateway into accessing all of the other ones.

- Scan your body from bottom to top. Turn your attention to relax each toe, ankle, calf, shin, knee, and thigh. Do this on the right side and on the left side, then take your attention to the hips, pelvis, groin. Work your way up to your belly, your chest, your rib cage, your back body, and the entire length of your spine. Let each point of focus be a cue for deeper rest and relaxation. Take time to linger through each point of focus so you allow ample time for each body part to find ease.

- Relax each of your fingers, your hands, your wrist, your forearm, your elbows, your upper arms, and your shoulders. Cue your armpits to surrender. Continue to take your awareness to your neck, your throat, your head, and your scalp.

- Gather a deep breath and exhale, allowing a wave of surrender to sweep over your body from head to toe.

- Now let your breath soften and become light and easy. Layer by layer, breath by breath, let go and rest for as long as you have time to do so.

- As you prepare to come to the end of your practice, circle your attention back to your intention. Chant it to yourself a few times and observe it rooting within you.

- Keeping your eyes closed, lazily bring yourself upright. Find an inner smile as you open your eyes.

Used with permission of Kali Alexander.

Avoiding Leg Cramps

Leg cramps can occur during your pregnancy, often when you sleep. Here are some tips to help prevent leg cramp (also known as charley horse).

- Stretch your calf muscles regularly. Down Dog is an easy and effective stretch. Drop your heels and lift your toes to deepen the stretch.

- Be sure to stay hydrated, as dehydration can increase the risk of cramping.

- Maintain electrolyte balance. If you are low in potassium, sodium, or magnesium, you might experience cramping.

- Choose good shoes with arch support.

Make Time for Exercise

You might be thinking, *Sleep is wonderful and self-care is important to me, but so is getting back into shape! Can you help rescue my figure?* Life does not stop and wait for us to get back into shape after having a baby, and whether it's a high school reunion or a baby shower, there is going to be an event that you would like to attend and feel comfortable in your body. I know, because this happened to me after my second baby was born. My 25th high school reunion was held two months to the day after my younger son was born. I knew I had to get back into shape quickly, to reflect my passion for fitness, and not show up as a sleepy hot mess. Reframing how you think of exercise can help you to give yourself permission to take time for self-care. We have all heard the expression "When mama isn't happy, no one is happy." You are the heart of the family, and keeping yourself happy and healthy as a mother is truly a gift to your family.

Over the years I have had to slim down for health and fitness DVDs, and I've helped celebrities get red carpet ready. I know quite a few techniques for getting in shape quickly when necessary. Full disclosure here: I was not always super healthy in the way that I used to get in shape fast. Before kids, I had quick tips and tricks that involved skipping meals, taking diuretics before photo shoots, and lots and lots of what I called *C+C*, which was caffeine and cardio. In the fitness industry, I have heard some pretty gross diets when folks are preparing for photo shoots. The worst I heard about was beef jerky and coffee. While it's really easy to judge that diet on so many levels, now that I am a little older, I can see where that instructor was desperate to get lean, and thought that desperate times called for desperate measures.

Rather than getting ready out of desperation or in a panicked way, you can actually have much better results by doing the work that you need to do to prepare, and then relax the day before your event. *Relax? Isn't that the opposite of what I need to do?* The truth is that stress can help us to pack on the weight and keep it on. When your nervous system goes into fight or flight mode, your adrenals pump out cortisol as a response to stress. Too much cortisol can lead to a number of physical changes, including rapid weight gain. How do you know when to work out and when to relax? Tables 11.1 to 11.3 provide basic schedules you can follow to get in shape fairly quickly, depending on how far out you are from your event. You might be surprised to see that there is a fair amount of rest, relaxation, and foam rolling involved. As crazy as it might sound, many women have better fat and weight loss results when there is a stress reduction plan in place.

In the world of exercise science there is a very effective approach to program design, called the *FITT Principle*. The initials stand for the four variables we can modify when creating your fitness program.

- Frequency
- Intensity
- Time (duration)
- Type

TABLE 11.1   SAMPLE WORKOUT SCHEDULE: TWO MONTHS BEFORE AN EVENT

	Sunday	Monday	Tuesday	Wednesday	Thursday	Friday	Saturday
a.m.	Walk 30 minutes	SOS practice	Walk 30 minutes	SOS practice	Walk 30 minutes	Yoga nidra	SOS practice
p.m.	Rescue Me practice	Walk 20 minutes	Rescue Me practice	Walk 20 minutes	Rescue Me practice	Rest	Rest

TABLE 11.2   SAMPLE WORKOUT SCHEDULE: TWO WEEKS BEFORE AN EVENT

	Sunday	Monday	Tuesday	Wednesday	Thursday	Friday	Saturday
a.m.	Walk 30 minutes wearing weighted vest	SOS practice	Walk 30 minutes wearing weighted vest	SOS practice	Walk 30 minutes wearing weighted vest	Yoga nidra	SOS practice
p.m.	Rescue Me practice	Walk 30 minutes wearing weighted vest	Rescue Me practice	Walk 30 minutes wearing weighted vest	Rescue Me practice	Rest	Rest

TABLE 11.3   SAMPLE WORKOUT SCHEDULE: TWO DAYS BEFORE AN EVENT

	Day 1	Day 2
a.m.	Walk uphill 15 minutes wearing weighted vest	Rest
p.m.	SOS practice	Yoga nidra

In the sample workouts provided, you will see that the frequency of your workout schedule is twice a day, as this is a great way to kick-start your program. The intensity in each workout is moderate, so that you don't burn out after the first few days. The duration of each workout is between 20 and 40 minutes, so that you average one hour of exercise a day, six days a week. The type of exercise is a combination of strength training, yoga, and cardio (walking). This particular program might be different from what you have done in the past, but I encourage you to try it when you need quick results. This training regimen is slow, steady, and consistent, which means that it is realistic that you can complete the eight weeks and meet your goals. My own goal is to set you up for success and to ease you into exercising moderately twice a day.

A Quick Note on Nutrition

We have addressed nutrition in previous chapters, but I know you might wonder whether you need different or additional information when you are preparing for an event. Following a balanced meal plan can help you regulate your weight. I do not recommend fad diets or extreme ways of eating. My key to being camera ready is to follow the old adage, "Eat breakfast like a king, lunch like a prince, and dinner like a pauper." Simply stated, make breakfast the largest meal of the day and try not to overeat at night. Staying on track with your nutrition will give you quicker results when you need to lean out for an event. One important point here is not just what you eat but what you drink too. It's really hard to get into killer shape if you are drinking soda, wine, or anything topped with whipped cream!

Recently, more and more moms are starting to drink cold-pressed juices, but be aware that many of these are high in sugar and calories. When purchasing juice, consider a vegetable-based juice so that your blood sugar does not spike. I would also recommend eating a handful of almonds at the same time, so that you also have some protein and fat to keep your blood sugar stable. Here are some easy tips to follow.

- Eat a large breakfast and a small dinner.
- Stay hydrated; it's easy to mistake thirst for hunger.
- Keep snacks handy; a small bag of trail mix can keep you from binging later.
- Stay accountable: Take photos of your meals throughout the day and review them at night.
- Try not to finish your children's food; those calories still count.
- Remember that food is fuel and not entertainment.
- Drink water, black coffee, or tea.

Athletes have a little-known secret called *two-a-days*, which simply refers to working out twice a day. I know that you are a busy mom and that trying to find the time for a second workout can be a challenge. That's why one of the workouts is walking, which can be done with your little one. Another acronym from exercise science is *EPOC* (excess postexercise oxygen consumption), known to trainers as *afterburn*. At the end of each exercise session there is a small window of time during which your body continues to burn fat and calories. The concept behind two-a-days is to take advantage of that window twice a day. Don't worry; you have a day off each week, and can adjust the schedule to fit your life.

The morning walks will help kick your metabolism into gear. You can start with brisk walking two months ahead of your event. When you are two weeks out from your event, I highly recommend baby wearing, if your little one weighs 20 pounds or less. If your little one is heavier than that, or prefers a stroller, you can wear a weighted vest while pushing the stroller. A 15-pound vest can be found on most online retailers; the price runs from around $20 for a plain one to $100 for a fancy one. There's really not much difference between them other than fashion.

Working out twice a day may sound like a lot at first, but if you have to get in shape quickly for an event, I can assure you that these types of workouts have brought my clients great success. It can take a few days to get into the rhythm of two separate exercise windows, but you will soon adjust and start to see results. There is no need to crash diet or punish yourself with grueling exercise. In fact, you might notice that you have more energy.

Yoga Poses and Exercises for Self-Care

The exercises in this book are designed to require minimal equipment. Your body weight is a great strength training tool, and you can do these exercises in the comfort of your own home, or at the gym. More often than not, your toddler will want to play with your stability ball and foam roller. Let your little one see you exercising and taking care of your body from the inside out. Your strong core can help you with everything from lifting baby to lifting the stroller into and out of the car.

When your baby starts to crawl is a great time to get in some extra core work. You will most likely spend hours a day sitting on the floor with your little one, playing and making them smile. Try to integrate a few of your own core strengthening moves during playtime. For example, you might hold Forearm Plank while your son or daughter starts to pull up to standing by using your shoulder or hip to steady themselves. In this way, you can both get stronger together. If you are enjoying yourself, your little one will see and feel that, and you can integrate a few strength moves into playtime.

Foam Roller for the Latissimus Dorsi

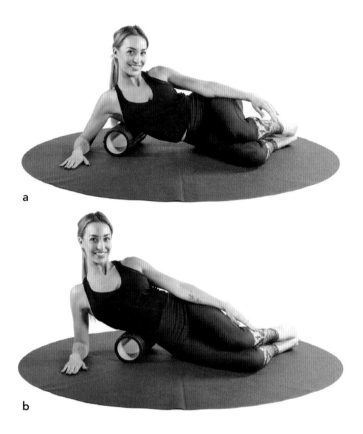

a

b

Benefits

This exercise releases tension in the fascia surrounding the latissimus dorsi muscles (lats) and helps with recovery.

Feeling

Enjoy the feeling of massage down the length of your lats. When you stand with your arms out to the sides, these muscles look like wings. Envision any heaviness dropping away from your wingspan as you roll away the tension.

Instruction

- Begin lying down on your right side with the foam roller beneath your armpit (see figure a). Extend your right arm straight alongside your ear, with the forearm on the floor.
- Place your left forearm on your left hip and slowly roll the foam roller from your armpit to just above your waist (see figure b), and then back up again.
- Repeat several times on the right, and then change sides.

Foam Roller for the Glutes

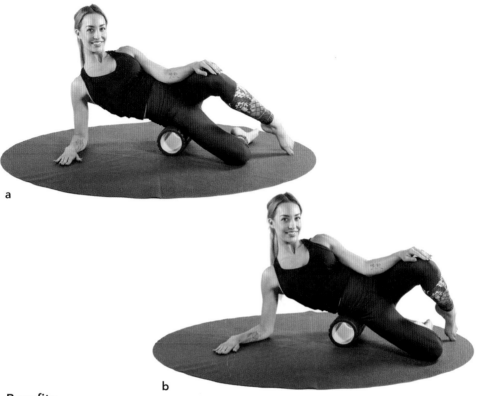

a

b

Benefits

This exercise releases tension in the fascia surrounding the glutes and helps with recovery.

Feeling

This usually gives the feeling we call *hurts so good*. The movement is a bit uncomfortable, very much like the discomfort of the first few moments of a shoulder massage.

Instruction

- Begin seated on the foam roller, with the roller wide (perpendicular to the length of your yoga mat).
- Cross your left ankle over your right calf, and place your left hand on your left knee. Rest your right hand in front of your right shoulder (see figure a).
- Slowly roll yourself forward (see figure b) and back on the foam roller. Take your time with this movement and if there is a spot that feels particularly tense, roll over that spot several times while breathing deeply.
- Repeat several times, and then switch sides.

Adjustments

If you prefer a more intense, deeper massage into your glutes, you can sit with the outer part of your glutes (the side of your bottom) on a tennis ball rather than on a foam roller. Slowly roll on the ball until you find a spot that is particularly tense, and with very small movements, roll back and forth on it.

Foam Roller for the IT Band

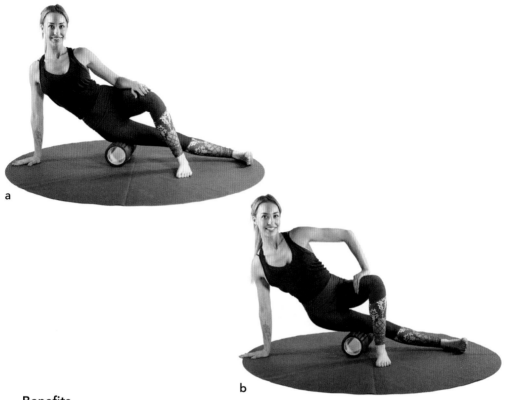

a

b

Benefits

This exercise releases tension in the fascia surrounding the IT band and helps with recovery.

Feeling

Foam rolling feels very much like a massage. Take your time with this exercise and enjoy some time dedicated to self-care.

Instruction

- Place the foam roller horizontally on your yoga mat about three quarters of the way back from the front of the mat.
- Sit with the bottom edge of your right outer hip on top of the foam roller and your right hand on the floor. Place your left foot in front of your right knee on the floor (see figure a).
- Slowly move your body so that the foam roller rolls down the length of your leg from the bottom of the hip to just above the knee (see figure b). Then roll from your knee to the top of the thigh.
- Move slowly and breathe deeply as you roll on the foam roller.

Adjustments

Bear in mind that a few rolls up and down the length of each leg is sufficient. Although this movement can feel a bit intense, a little bit goes a long way. Take your time and listen to your body.

Fish Pose on Foam Roller

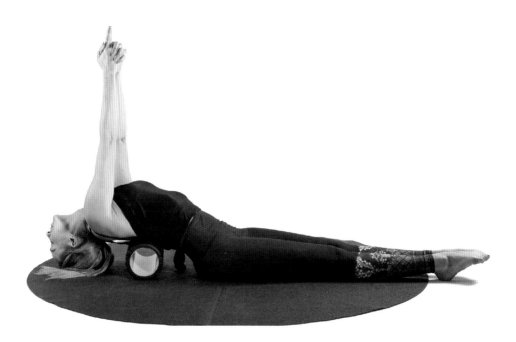

Benefits

This exercise stretches the chest and abdominal muscles and lengthens them.

Feeling

The chest rises to the sky as though it were the back of a fish. If you practice the variation with the arms reaching out toward the sky, your arms take the shape of the fish's fin. Stay playful with your attitude and envision the fish whose shape you are creating.

Instruction

- Begin seated on the floor with your legs extended straight in front of you and the foam roller behind your hips.
- Slowly bring your hands behind the foam roller and begin to lie down on your back. Adjust the foam roller so that it is directly under your shoulder blades (see figure). The classical pose is practiced with the arms extended to the sky, the fingers interlaced, and the index fingers extended up.
- Breathe slowly, deeply, and mindfully.

Adjustments

For an easier variation, simply keep your arms at your sides and your hands on the floor.

Burpee

Benefits

The Burpee is a total body exercise. It provides muscle strengthening and cardiovascular work along with core work.

Feeling

In kundalini yoga, there is a series of movements called *kriya*. Similar to Burpees, it is said to help purify anger: When you push the body physically, you take the fight out of the body. When you take the fight out of the body, you also take the fight out of the mind. In this way, anger begins to subside. Use Burpees to help you relieve stress while also working your muscles, joints, and heart in a positive way.

Instruction

▌ Begin standing tall with your feet hip width apart (see figure a).

▌ Lower your hips into a deep squat and place your hands on the floor (see figure b).

▌ Jump back to the bottom of a push-up (see figure c).

▌ From the push-up position, look forward to your hands and jump your feet into a squat with your hands still on the floor (see figure d).

▌ Explosively jump straight up with your arms overhead (see figure e) and repeat from the beginning.

Adjustments

If you are not comfortable jumping back or forward, it's OK to step back to a push-up position and then step forward to standing. Note that if you are choosing to step front and back, make sure to alternate the foot that you lead with each time, so as to maintain balance from right to left.

a

b

c

d

e

Alternating Reverse Lunge

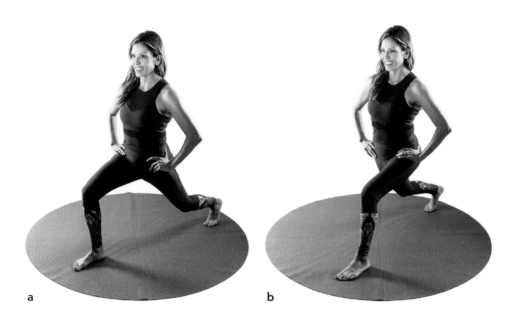

a   b

Benefits

This exercise strengthens the lower body.

Feeling

Alternating Reverse Lunges are challenging. Know that the challenge is empowering you with strength, and remember that you are getting stronger with each repetition.

Instruction

- Begin standing with your feet hip width apart and your hands on your hips.
- As you inhale, step your left foot back into a Lunge position with the right (front) knee at a 90 degree angle (see figure a). Your right knee will almost touch the floor. Make sure that your upper body stays upright and that you engage your core muscles.
- Exhale as you return to the start position. Alternate sides (see figure b).

Adjustments

This exercise can be made more challenging by adding weight. Dumbbells in your hands or a barbell across your upper back and shoulders will increase the amount of work for your upper body and will elevate your heart rate as well. You can also add upper body training by performing a biceps curl as you step back into the lunge.

Modified Handstand

Benefits

The handstand helps you to develop total body strength because it requires coordination, stability, and strengthening in each position.

Feeling

Inversions bring the head below the heart and give a different perspective of the world. Enjoy seeing things from your new view and remember that seeing life from many different perspectives can often bring new insight.

Instruction

- Begin standing with your back approximately 12 inches away from a wall.
- Hinge from the hips to move into a Forward Fold, with your hands on the floor, shoulder width apart. Walk one foot up the wall behind you, and then the other, until your body is at a 90 degree angle with your hands shoulder-width apart (see figure a).
- Slowly climb your feet up the wall until your legs are straight. If you would like more of a challenge, slowing lift your right leg straight up to the sky for 3 to 5 breaths, then change sides (see figure b).
- Breathe deeply, and when you are ready to dismount, slowly lower one foot to the floor, and then the other, and you can end in the starting position of a Forward Fold.

Adjustments

If it's too scary to walk your legs all the way up at first, just go as far as you feel comfortable. That's OK; it's natural to protect our vital organs (our brain and our heart). You can try to walk the feet up the wall until your body is at a 90 degree angle (see figure a). You will develop strength and balance in the modification, so it's a great place to begin.

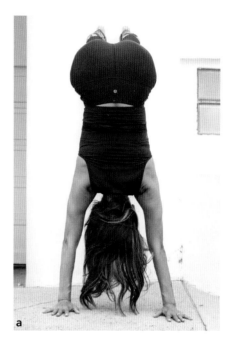

a

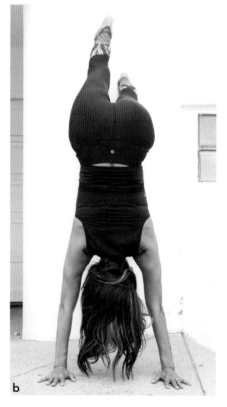

b

Straight Leg Crunch With Hip Raise

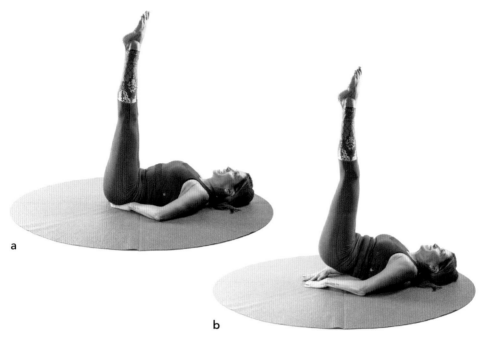

a

b

Benefits

This exercise strengthens the core, with a focus on the lower fibers of the TVA and the abs.

Feeling

Imagine that there is an X on the ceiling and that you're trying to press your feet onto the X. The X should be directly over your hips, not over your face. This simple visualization will help you execute the exercise correctly as you lift your lower body toward the X.

Instruction

- Begin lying down on your back with your legs straight up in the air at a 90 degree angle (see figure a). Place your hands flat on the floor under your glutes with your palms facing down.
- Slowly lift your hips and legs straight up toward the ceiling, taking care to make sure that your ankles, knees, and hips are all in alignment (see figure b). Be aware that the motion should feel like gliding, and not like jumping abruptly with the lower body.

Adjustments

If this is a newer exercise for you, it can help to have someone hold your legs between their arms, ensuring that your legs are in line with your hips and not moving back toward your face. Or you can do this exercise next to a mirror to make sure that you are doing it correctly. As with most exercises, a slight bend in the knee will take pressure off of the lower back. You can also use a folded blanket under your lower back for added support.

Chaturanga Pose

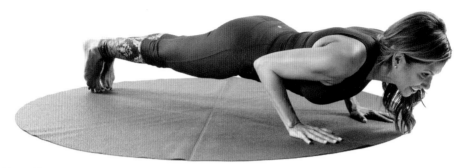

Benefits

This pose strengthens the pecs, triceps, and core stabilizers.

Feeling

The Spanish word for push-up is *lagartija*, which means lizard. At the bottom of the movement, allow your body to hover above the floor like a lizard. Try to stay playful with your approach and light with your attitude.

Instruction

- Begin in Plank Position (top of a push-up) with your hands shoulder width apart.
- Engage your core muscles and exhale as you slowly bend your elbows and keep your torso hovering above the floor (see figure). Make sure that your spine stays long and your gaze can remain slightly forward, approximately 12 inches ahead of the front of your yoga mat.
- You can repeat this exercise for several repetitions by straightening the arms, or you can enjoy the movement as part of a flow sequence.

Adjustments

You can bring your knees to the floor into modified Chaturanga (see chapter 4). By taking your knees to the floor you are working with less resistance, and the exercise is less challenging.

Putting It All Together

Taking care of your body is integral to your ability to feel energized each morning. Working out hard is not always what the body needs. If you have a big event coming up, remember that rest is an integral part of muscle repair. Tight, tense muscles can benefit greatly from the Rescue Me practice. If on the other hand you know that it is time to kick your program into high gear (your body is healed from childbirth, you have proper rest, and have your doctor's clearance), then the SOS practice can help you to burn calories and sculpt your body. An easy way to test what you need is to go for a 20 minute walk every other day (at least 3 months postpartum), and see how you feel at the end of the walk. If you are feeling depleted and drained, pull out your foam roller and enjoy some self-care time. If you are feeling energized and ready for more, choose the SOS workout. Remember to stay receptive to the feedback of your body, exercise should never be a form of punishment.

Having a baby and becoming a mom requires a lot of lifting, stretching, and physical work. Some days the body needs more of a work in than a work-out. This practice is intended for those who are at least six to eight weeks postpartum, or whenever you have clearance from your doctor.

Turning your attention inward and taking the time to massage tired muscles and tense connective tissue can feel fantastic. This workout is designed to give you the feeling of massage from the inside out. Note that a foam roller and a yoga mat are needed for this practice.

Exercise	Page	Focus	Reps/Time
Child's Pose	59	Stretches the lower back and hips; invites ease	3-5 slow, deep, centering breaths focusing on the inhalation and the exhalation being equal in length
Unicorn and Rainbow Pose	52	Lower back, abdomen	5 rounds; it's OK to gently tuck the tailbone now that you are postpartum
Foam Roller for the Spine	166	Muscles that support the spine	60-90 seconds on your back
Foam Roller for the Latissimus Dorsi	236	Lats	60-90 seconds on right and left
Foam Roller for the Glutes	237	Glutes	60-90 seconds on right and left
Foam Roller for the IT Band	238	IT band	60-90 seconds on the side of your upper thighs
Fish Pose on the Foam Roller	239	Chest, abdomen	5-9 breaths
Deep Relaxation Pose	66	Entire body	1-3 minutes

SOS: POSTPARTUM QUICK-START PRACTICE

Sometimes we need a quick start to get in shape for a particular event. If you need to get in shape fairly quickly but don't have a lot of time, this workout program will help you to tone up. This practice is intended for those who are at least 3 or 4 months postpartum, or whenever you have your doctor's clearance. The exercises and yoga postures are intended to work your body as a whole, so take your time with this workout and take breaks in between sets so that you can give each exercise one hundred percent.

Exercise	Page	Focus	Reps/Time
Half Sun Salutation	48	Shoulders, core strength and flexibility	3 rounds; remember that each movement corresponds to an inhalation or exhalation
Sun Salutation B	80	Entire body	3 rounds; remember that each movement corresponds to an inhalation or exhalation
Burpee	240	Entire body	3 sets of 5-8 reps
Alternating Reverse Lunge	241	Lower body	2-3 sets of 10-12 reps right and left
Chaturanga Pose	244	Chest, triceps, shoulders	3 sets of 5-8 reps

Exercise	Page	Focus	Reps/Time
Modified Handstand	242	Chest, triceps, shoulders, core	3-5 deep breaths when you feel confident in your handstand
Straight Leg Crunch With Hip Raise	243	Core muscles	3 sets of 10-15 reps
Supine Hand-to-Big-Toe Pose with a Twist	168	Outer thighs and hips	5-9 breaths on the right and left
Deep Relaxation Pose	66	Entire body	1-3 minutes

*M*ommy Move

Lateral Raise

If you know you have an event coming up in the next few months, one of the easiest exercises you can do to help look great quickly is a Lateral Raise. Lateral Raises train your shoulder muscles, specifically the medial deltoid, or side of the shoulder. This exercise can give you definition in the upper arm and help your entire upper body look fit. Also, when you train the shoulder muscles and put a small amount of muscle mass on the shoulders, it gives the illusion of making the waist look smaller, much like shoulder pads did in the 1980s.

For this exercise you will need handheld weights that are between 5 and 10 pounds each. If you do not have weights, you can substitute a heavy household item, such as two bottles of laundry detergent (making sure to keep them out of the reach of children). Begin with your feet hip width apart and a slight bend in your knees. Stand up tall with your core naturally engaged and, as you exhale, lift your arms out to the side with a soft, natural bend at the elbow. Pause when your hands are just below the height of your shoulders, and slowly lower as you inhale. Do 12 to 15 reps, and notice the natural tone in your shoulders at the top of the movement. The goal is to train the shoulders to look this way even when you are not lifting weights.

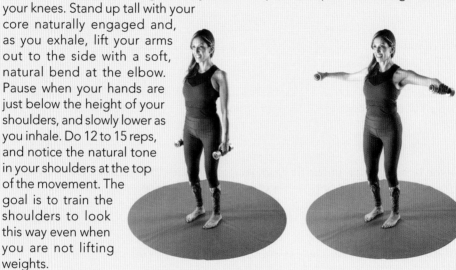

*I*nformation No One Tells You

A Cheat Meal Can Increase Your Sex Drive

What we do most of the time has the greatest impact on our health and wellness. If we are exercising and eating healthy 95 percent of the week, it is more than OK to have a cheat meal; in fact, some experts recommend it. Here are a few of the reasons a cheat meal can be beneficial.

▌ A cheat meal can prevent you from feeling deprived (psychological benefit).

▌ A cheat meal can help to move you past a weight-loss plateau (physical benefit).

▌ An increase in leptin, specifically from carbs, can help increase your sex drive (physiological benefit). Leptin is a hormone that helps control hunger, appetite, and libido. A prolonged calorie-restricted diet can lower leptin levels, which can lead to an underactive libido and sex drive. (Your sex drive might be a little low anyway from lack of sleep.)

For my private clients, I recommend one high-carb cheat meal per week to help kick everything into gear: your metabolism, your sunny outlook, and your sex drive. Be aware that it is only one meal per week and not a whole day of binging. That one meal can be whatever you might be craving, even pizza.

Love-Your-Baby Visualization

Awakening Kundalini Shakti

Kundalini yoga was introduced to the West by Yogi Bhajan, and incorporates the idea of coiled feminine energy at the base of the spine. The idea is that untapped potential is latent in our first three chakras (root, sacral, and solar plexus), and that we can invite that energy to rise and help us realize that untapped potential. Yes, it sounds pretty far out there, but the way something sounds and the way it feels can often be worlds apart. This practice can help you feel that your life force energy is reawakening, sort of like a reboot for your physical body. I encourage you to take a chance with this visualization and notice how it makes you feel. Note that kundalini yoga, like all yoga, is not a religion. The kriya techniques involve internal and external movements to help awaken your body's own life force, and are completely safe.

Begin seated in a comfortable cross-legged position with a meditation cushion or pillow beneath your sit bones for support. Sit up tall and elongate your neck. Visualize your root chakra as a strong grounding cord, rooting your energy in Mother Earth. Now slowly begin to circle your upper body in a Sufi Roll (see chapter 10). You can envision a spiral of energy dancing around your spine, looking much like the double helix of DNA, as you continue to circle the upper body. Sense, see, and feel the energy begin to rise up from your lower back to your middle back. Notice the feeling of energy rising within you, as though someone has turned on all the lights in the house of your body. Little by little, sense this energy rising up to your upper back, and continue to see the double helix of light dancing around your spine. Allow this energy to rise to the base of your neck, to your head, and finally to the crown of your head and beyond. Continue to sit and breathe as you feel the energy rising from the base of the spine to the crown and note any images or ideas that come to your mind. When you feel a sense of completion, slowly open your eyes, and journal any new ideas that came to mind.

Fun Foods

While working out at Gold's Gym Venice, California (aka the mecca of bodybuilding), I met an amazing female bodybuilder named Shannan Yorton Penna. Shannan created the popular Quest bars that you see on the market, and her delicious recipes leave you very satisfied. Here is her recipe for protein pizza.

Protein Pizza Crust
Contributed by Shannan Yorton Penna

      1 cup shredded mozzarella cheese

      1/2 cup shredded parmesan cheese

      2 ounces cream cheese

      3/4 cup blanched almond flour

      1 large egg

> continued

Preheat oven to 425°. Combine mozzarella, parmesan, and cream cheese in a microwaveable bowl and microwave for 30 seconds. Take out of microwave and stir. Microwave for another 30 seconds and stir again. Add the almond flour and the egg. Mix with a fork until the ingredients combine and begin to cool. Then knead by hand and form into a pizza crust on a nonstick pan. (It can be difficult to shape the crust by hand; it helps place parchment paper over the crust and roll with a rolling pin.) You can also cut the crust to individual sizes or shapes with a knife or a large cookie cutter. Bake for 12 to14 minutes until it's done just the way you like it: crispy brown or just lightly golden. Remove from the oven, add desired toppings, and bake for an additional 5 to 7 minutes.
Yield: one pizza

Insights
for Moms Over 40

Advanced maternal age used to be the term for women who were pregnant over the age of 35. Today's term is *geriatric*, which makes us sound and feel ancient. I had my first baby at the age of 37 and was considered high risk. My doctor explained to me that I was incredibly healthy, but that I would be sent to a high-risk specialist because of my age. The high-risk specialist told me that my pregnancy was normal and healthy and not to worry. I never imagined I would see that same doctor again at age 42 with my second pregnancy. Both pregnancies were planned, but I had never thought I'd be pregnant again in my 40s. The day I delivered our second baby, I couldn't help but wonder if I was the oldest mom at the hospital. I asked the labor and delivery nurse if I was indeed the oldest mom they had ever seen, and she giggled and said, "Not by a long shot."

Women are having babies well into their late 40s; my doula recently helped a 52-year-old mom through a happy, healthy pregnancy. With women having babies later in life, it is important to look at some of the unique challenges that come with advanced maternal age. Call me old school, but I still can't use the term *geriatric*. Some women have fertility issues later in life and need some help getting pregnant, often through IVF. Even when there are no fertility issues, it can be a bit more of a challenge to get back into shape, simply because our metabolism slows down a little over the age of 35. However, there are some incredibly inspiring women who reclaim their strength after pregnancy later in life; I invited two such women to share their stories in this chapter.

Age really *is* just a number and we can all strive to be the healthiest, best versions of ourselves at any age. Sometimes clients assume that I am naturally fit and that I don't have to work for it. I am 46, with a thyroid condition and two children who were both born after I was 36. I know that you can get back into great shape after having babies later in life because I did it, and I am surrounded by more and more women who are doing this every day. It's said that age brings wisdom, and we learn to become more discerning in life, and that includes our workouts. Gone are the days of liquid diets, binge exercising, and guilt cycles that come with overeating and punishing workouts. Balanced exercise, balanced eating, and a healthy relationship with exercise, food, and our own bodies can help transform how we see ourselves.

Your Body Over 40

Over the age of 40, changes occur in a woman's body. With these changes comes an increased risk of certain conditions including preeclampsia, gestational diabetes, preterm delivery, and problems with the placenta. While most women who are pregnant in their 30s and 40s go on to have normal pregnancies, it is the responsibility of your health care professional to inform you about the risks.

Your Hormones and Your Age

Hormonal balance is an important topic during pregnancy and beyond. In our 40s we also notice slight shifts in hormone levels at perimenopause and during menopause itself. Here is a basic guide to understanding the function of our hormones.

- *Human chorionic gonadotropin (HCG)* is produced by what becomes the placenta. When you take a home pregnancy test, you are testing for the presence of HCG. HCG affects the ovaries by pausing ovulation throughout pregnancy, essentially telling your body that it is pregnant.
- *Progesterone* relaxes smooth muscle tissue, including the wall of the uterus. Progesterone enriches the uterus with a thick lining of blood cells to support the health of the growing fetus. This relaxing of smooth muscle tissue affects digestion and can often lead to constipation during pregnancy. Progesterone also helps the mother's body to tolerate foreign DNA (from the fetus).
- *Estrogen* stimulates hormone production in the baby's adrenal gland and enhances the mother's uterus, which allows the uterus to respond to oxytocin. Estrogen levels decline during menopause.
- *Oxytocin* is said to trigger labor (much like Pitocin, the synthetic form of oxytocin). Oxytocin stretches the cervix for labor and delivery and allow the breasts to produce milk after baby is born.
- *Prolactin* is the hormone that prepares the breasts to produce milk; it is said to have a tranquilizing effect.
- *Relaxin* loosens and relaxes the ligaments in preparation for labor and delivery so that your baby can pass through your pelvis.

Maternal Heart Rate

Your heart has to work harder during pregnancy because as the fetus grows the heart has to pump more blood to the uterus. As a result of this extra work, your resting heart rate will increase from about 70 beats per minute prepregnancy to as much as 80 to 90 beats per minute during pregnancy. Years ago, the indication for pregnant women was not to let the heart rate get higher than 140 beats per minute during exercise. That number is not used as commonly today since there is such a wide array of cardiovascular

In the fitness industry, a few incredibly fit women are well known for specific body parts. In the late 1990s, a woman named Theresa Hessler (now Sauter) was known for her abs and frequently graced the pages of many national fitness magazines. In 2012, while training at Gold's Gym, I met Theresa, who was pregnant with her first daughter. I recognized her as the model with the incredible abs, and I soon found out that her beautifully fierce spirit is even stronger than her core muscles. I learned that she had had a long and challenging road with fertility and with fitness. Theresa is an inspiration to me; she has shown me what true perseverance and inner strength are all about. Every time we speak, she reminds me how truly strong women are. Here is her story as told to me.

Desi: *Tell me about your journey to becoming a mom.*

Theresa: *My journey to becoming a mom was met with many challenges. It started with me finding the right man and getting married at the age of 40. We started trying to conceive as soon as we were married. It didn't take long to see a positive pregnancy test. Disappointingly, that was short lived, as the pregnancy ended as a chemical pregnancy. I was about to discover that this was only the beginning of a very long and exhausting journey. After two years of fertility treatments, and lots of fertility drugs, and four miscarriages, we took a break. While I was on break, I became pregnant naturally with my oldest daughter Chloe. She was a miracle according to my doctor. A year after Chloe's birth, we decided we wanted one more child to complete our family. We immediately decided on egg donation because we knew at age 44 the odds of fertility treatments working were not in our favor. Our donor cycle produced 13 genetically normal embryos. We thought pregnancy would be a slam dunk after our first transfer. Unfortunately, that was not the case. After four more miscarriages, I found myself on more fertility drugs than when I had been trying to conceive with my own eggs. My sixth transfer produced a successful pregnancy. A healthy baby girl was born as a result. However, it left me with a hefty price to pay: my health.*

Desi: *Tell me more about your health.*

Theresa: *Health and fitness is my passion. It has always been a part of me from a very young age. I worked out up until the day that I delivered my first child. However, with my second, I found that I did not feel well most of the pregnancy. After the delivery of my second child, I discovered that I was very sick. My blood pressure shot up to 180/110, my cholesterol was high, there were blood sugar issues, adrenal fatigue, hypothyroidism, digestive issues, thrush, yeast infections, and eventually a cancer diagnosis. I knew that I needed to take action quickly. The doctor wanted to prescribe a myriad of pharmaceutical drugs. However, I knew that putting a Band-Aid on the situation with drugs was not a solution to help me heal long term. I needed to get to the root of the problem. I have always been more holistic, plus after all of the fertility drugs, I felt that pharmaceuticals were something I should leave as a last resort.*

Desi: *Tell me about your postpartum physical recovery and exercise. Were you able to work out?*

Theresa: *After I delivered Maddy, I was pretty sick. I think that all of the fertility drugs took a toll, and my daughter was not sleeping at night, so I really had to change things up a lot. I was told that I should really take it easy, so for my fitness program, I started out with just 10 minutes a day. I started exercising around the house doing squats, lunges, push-ups, planks,*

> continued

Theresa's Story > *continued*

and exercises that used my body weight. Soon thereafter, I then started a few rounds of high-intensity intervals to get my heart rate up, but I started to notice that I was feeling fatigued, and almost like I was getting the flu. I really had to be careful about how much I did.

I suspect that a lot of women in my age category who have gone through multiple fertility treatments have had a similar experience with all of the drugs taking a toll on your body. For me, I returned to fitness slowly, and I would exercise in 10-minute windows and then see how I felt the next day. If I did not feel good the next day, I would take the day off. Eventually I was able to build up to 20 minutes, and then 30 minutes, simply by listening to my body. It's been two and a half years now, and I am just now getting to the point where I can go to the gym and do a workout and feel OK the next day. It was a long road back.

Desi: *What has helped you recover your energy and strength?*

Theresa: *For me, things shifted when I started to realign my circadian rhythm. I have learned that a lot of things can be corrected by getting cortisol levels back into balance. My cortisol levels were off largely because of the lack of sleep from being up all night and breastfeeding every couple of hours. Like for so many other moms, getting up in the middle of the night can be hard. Waking up when it is still dark out is not natural, and so I bought a light box. I started using the light box in the morning to pick up my cortisol levels. In my personal research, I have found that going back to basics really helps to heal your body. You do not need a bunch of supplements or drugs to get back into rhythm. The best way to get back into rhythm is to wake up when the sun rises, and if that is not possible, then the light box can really help.*

Used with permission of Theresa Sauter.

fitness levels, and heart rate tests are not one-size-fits-all. Today, trainers and instructors are more likely to use the talk test with pregnant women. The talk test is exactly what it sounds like: You should be able to speak a few sentences without feeling or sounding winded. If you feel you cannot speak comfortably, you are likely working too hard.

Exercise Over 40

After the age of 35 our metabolism slows down, and what worked for maintenance in the past is no longer enough. Slow weight gain might steadily creep up in the form of 1 or 2 pounds a year. This doesn't sound like much until, 10 years later, nothing in your closet fits. Taking the time to add a little extra cardiovascular exercise, and taking the long way when walking home can help increase your ability to maintain the weight at which you feel comfortable. It is not always necessary to do more exercises. Instead, try exercising more often (six days a week if you can), increase the intensity in a moderate way by carrying light hand weights, increase the length of your walking by five minutes a day, and of course cross-train.

Also, in working with thousands of women over the years, I have found that many women, including myself, lose some tone in their derriere during pregnancy. The booty gets a little bigger with the extra weight from pregnancy, but then after baby is born, it can feel as though your bottom fell down. This can also happen as we get a little bit older; we lose muscle mass and some of the strength and tone in the glutes. Squatting and lunging are my favorite lower body exercises. Lunges, sometimes called split squats, are incredibly effective in helping to increase strength and definition in your legs and glutes. Both of these exercises are portable; you can do them anywhere, at any time, with no equipment other than your own body weight.

Squatting is a type of movement that you will see in almost every form of exercise. Our bodies are designed to bend at the knees and at the hips. There are many types of squats: sumo squats (aka plié), plyometric squats, single leg squats (aka lunges), goblet squats; the list goes on. Squatting has many benefits, which include strengthening the glutes, quadriceps, hamstrings, calves, and core muscles. In the world of physical therapy, doctors refer to these muscles as the posterior chain. It is common for the posterior chain to be somewhat neglected because as a society we have a tendency to sit a lot and because it's natural to train the muscles that we can see in the mirror.

Moms benefit from posterior training during pregnancy and after baby is born. During pregnancy, there is a shift in the center of gravity, in addition to the weight of the beautiful baby pulling the belly forward. All of this leads to a tense lower back and a weak posterior chain, unless you are training. Additionally, after baby is born, there is a lot of sitting and holding baby on one hip. Several imbalances can occur between your abdominals, hip flexors, hamstrings, and lower back. Training your glutes correctly can help to correct some of these muscular imbalances that can so commonly occur. A few posterior chain exercises that can help balance your strength, and ultimately your posture as well, include squats, lunges, deadlifts, glute bridges, and hip extensions, all of which are included later in this chapter.

With exercises overlapping, and so many that look the same from one system of movement to another, you might be wondering, *What is the best type of exercise?* The best answer I have ever heard was from my friend and former Miss Olympia competitor, Joanne Lee Cornish, who said, "The best type of exercise is the exercise that you will do." Finding a form of movement that you enjoy can be just as important as the benefits of that type of movement. Joy will keep you in it for the long haul, and can benefit your body, mind, and spirit. I love yoga and fitness, and see the benefits in both. When a movement does not feel great for one of my clients, I have a separate set of tools I can draw from. The joy of movement comes in many different formats: yoga, fitness, dance, Pilates, walking, indoor cycling, HIIT training, and much more. Look for similarities in the various systems of movement; in the movements that overlap in various systems, you will see the ways the body is designed to move. Our bodies are clearly designed to squat, stand, bend over, twist, walk, push, and pull.

In the late 1990s, I lived in Cabo San Lucas, Mexico, where I owned a small health and fitness studio. At that time, very few American fitness publications were available at the local store, but they always had *Oxygen* magazine. One article described a model who embodied strength and grace and looked like she had amazing energy. I cut out her picture and put it on my refrigerator. That model was Amy Fadhli.

Fast-forward to 2017, when I met Amy Fadhli Raymond at Gold's Gym in Venice, California. I had to tell her that she used to be on my fridge. I now work out with her husband, Tito Raymond, and have gotten to know Amy. She is an incredibly inspiring woman who underwent fertility treatments in her 40s to create the beautiful, healthy family she has today. Here is her story and her fitness tips for moms.

Being a pregnant woman of advanced maternal age (I was 40 when I had my first child), I was told to take it easy during my pregnancy, not just because of my age, but also because I had done in vitro for both pregnancies. I waited until the embryo was vital (first heartbeat at six weeks), then I started gradually reintroducing and implementing my training regimen. This included daily resistance training as well as cardio workouts on the stationary bike, elliptical, the treadmill, and the giant StepMill. The main limitation I had for myself was to make sure my heart rate did not exceed 140 bpm, as was suggested by my ob/gyn. I realize that this recommendation has changed somewhat, but 12 years ago, this was still recommended. I also did not do abdominal exercises. What's the point, I thought, and my fertility doctor advised against it as he thought my midsection needed to relax a bit for the pregnancy.

However, with all the squatting and lunging and athletic moves, I was keeping my core engaged and staying somewhat fit in the midsection. This would prove to be advantageous after the delivery via C-section of both my children! In order to keep my heart rate down below 140, I had to lower the amounts of my weights. For instance, instead of squatting 125 pounds, I could only do 100 to 105. And the intensity with which I trained was quite a bit slower. I had to rest a little bit longer in between each set just to make sure I wasn't overexerting.

For my first pregnancy, I only gained 28 pounds and the second one (three and a half years later) I gained about 31 pounds. I still ate healthily and fairly clean because that's my taste. But if I had a craving, I satiated it! Postpregnancy recovery was much easier than I was led to believe. Having had C-sections for both pregnancies, I was profoundly aware of the possibility of scar tissue inhibiting activities. So I made sure that I started walking the hospital hallways while pushing the bassinet after the first day. When I got home after being in the hospital for 3 or 4 days, I started going on power walks with the stroller and that seemed to help my recovery a lot!

I had no problems with recovery, and within two weeks I was back in the gym, taking it easy of course. Within six weeks post-C-section I was able to start doing a little bit of abdominal work like planking and light crunches. I actually feel like training my abs helped break up the scar tissue that inevitably forms after a C-section.

Yoga Poses and Exercises for Moms Over 40

They say that age brings wisdom. In my experience, it also brings a lot of insight into how our individual body works when we are in our 40s. After living in your body for 40 years, you probably have a clear idea of what your body likes to do and what makes it thrive. Included here are some of my favorite exercises for pre- and postnatal fitness in your 40s.

Squat

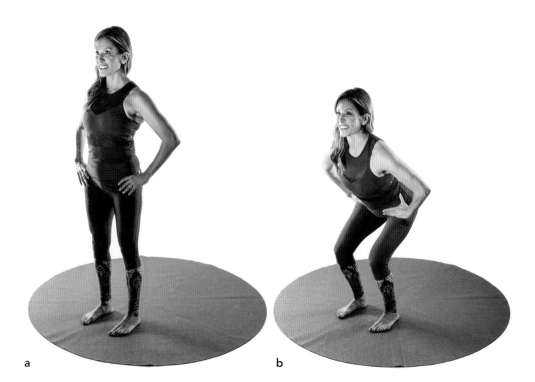

a

b

Benefit

This exercise strengthens the entire body, with emphasis on the lower body, especially the glutes, hamstrings, quads, and TVA.

Feeling

Squats are all about lower body strength. Feel the power in your legs, glutes, and core. This movement is reminiscent of the position that athletes perform all the time. Everyone from jockeys to ice hockey players squats for a position of power. Take inspiration from your favorite sport and remember that you are an athlete.

Instruction

- Stand with your feet hip width apart, toes pointed straight ahead (see figure a).
- Inhale as you lower your bottom as though you were going to sit in a chair, hands on your hips (see figure b).
- Exhale as you slowly straighten your legs and return to standing. Make sure to keep your core engaged throughout the exercise.

Adjustments

This exercise can be done with a chair behind your bottom so that you have a tactile cue as to how deep your squat should be. Each time you squat, gently tap your bottom on the chair so that you reach the optimal level of depth.

Firedancer Squat

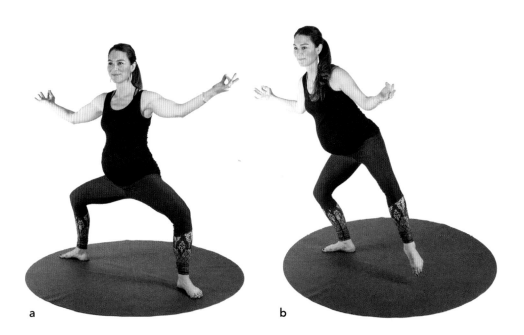

a   b

Benefits

This exercise strengthens the entire lower body with emphasis on the quadriceps, glutes, and pelvic floor muscles.

Feeling

If you have ever watched Hawaiian fire dancers in a deep squat, with palm leaves around their wrists or ankles, you know the image of them squatting in their power. They look connected to Mother Earth even when lifting a foot of the floor. Feel the power in your lower body and envision a grounding cord moving from the base of your spine to the earth.

Instruction

- Begin by standing up tall with your feet hip width apart and your core lightly engaged.
- Slowly bend your knees and draw your hips back into a squat position, keeping the chest upright (see figure a).
- Exhale and rise halfway up to straight legs while lifting your left foot (see figure b).
- Inhale and return to the squat position with both feet on the floor.
- Exhale and rise halfway up to straight legs while lifting your left foot.
- Continue the exercise, alternating sides.

Adjustments

If maintaining the lower squat is too intense or challenging, it's OK to come up to completely straight legs between squats.

Squat Jump

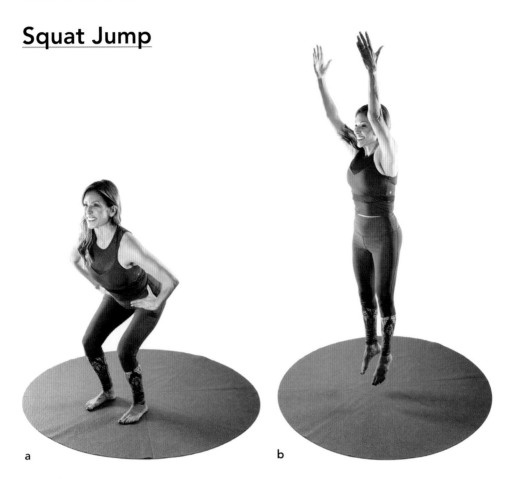

a   b

Benefits

This exercise strengthens the entire body, with emphasis on the lower body, especially the glutes, hamstrings, quads, and TVA.

Feeling

The feeling of the exercise is strong and explosive. Rather than attacking the movement, think of it as a game. Small children often try to jump up to touch the ceiling or the top of a basketball rim. Find a visual cue at least three feet above your head that you can aim for, and reach for it each time. Have fun with it!

Instruction

- Stand with your feet hip width apart, toes pointed straight ahead.
- Inhale as you lower your bottom as though you were going to sit in a chair, hands on your hips (see figure a).
- Exhale as you jump straight up in the air while reaching overhead (see figure b). Keep your core engaged as you jump up.

Adjustments

You can make this exercise as big and explosive as you like. Adjust the tempo to find a rhythm that allows for several repetitions so that you feel challenged but not winded.

Jumping Lunge

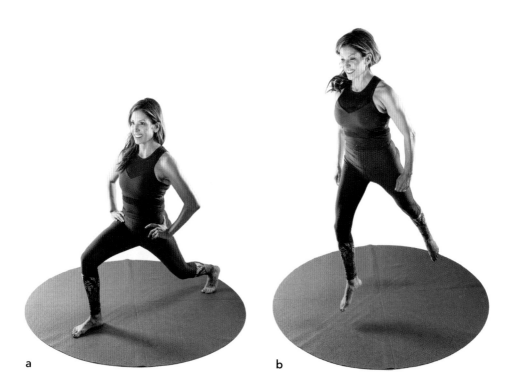

a

b

Benefits

This exercise increases cardiovascular endurance while strengthening the lower body.

Feeling

This exercise looks and feels like a photo of Michael Jordan shooting a basket. The idea is that you are trying to get some hang time in the air and land gracefully each time. Think of someone who inspires you—perhaps a famous ice skater or basketball player—who achieves power while jumping. Those with athletic prowess have a certain grace, making their landing look effortless.

Instruction

- Begin with your feet hip width apart and your core engaged.
- Place your hands on your hips and jump your left leg back into a lunge with your right knee at a 90 degree angle (see figure a).
- Jump back up and switch your legs in midair, making sure you keep your chest upright throughout (see figure b).

Adjustments

To make the move more explosive, you can use your arms as if running, to help you power up as your legs switch. Repeat.

Running Man

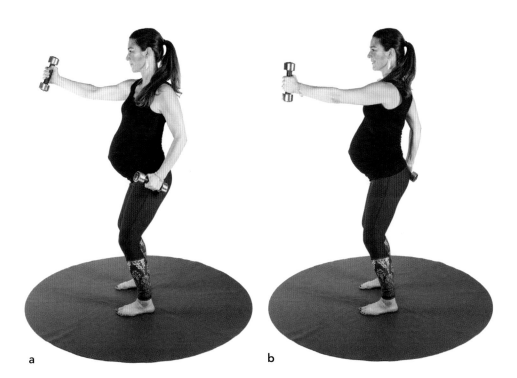

a   b

Benefits

This exercise strengthens the shoulders while lightly engaging the core muscles.

Feeling

As the name indicates, this movement is reminiscent of the arm motion while running; there is a natural rhythm to the alternating lift.

Instruction

- Stand with your feet hip width apart and a soft bend in your knees.
- While holding a dumbbell in each hand, slowly lift your right hand up to 90 degrees (shoulder level) while extending the left arm back to a degree that feels safe for you.
- Change sides and now lift the left arm while extending the right arm behind you.
- Continue to alternate while breathing deeply.

Adjustments

To make the exercise less challenging, sit on a weight training bench or folding chair with your feet and knees hip width apart. The support under your hips will make the exercise easier for your core, and it feels good on the days that your pelvis feels heavy, especially in the third trimester.

Warrior 3 Pose With Hands on Wall

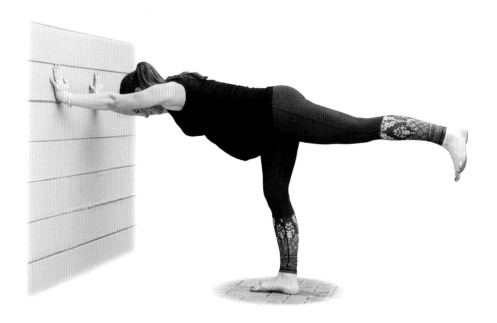

Benefits

This pose strengthens the stabilizers of the standing leg and the hamstring of the lifted leg. It also lightly engages the abs and the obliques.

Feeling

The feeling in Warrior 3 is that of driving forward. After the warrior has risen from the earth (Warrior 1), he draws his sword (Warrior 2), and charges forward as he strikes (Warrior 3). As you charge forward into motherhood, feel your strength and power, the power of a mother.

Instruction

- Begin standing facing a wall and walk your feet back until your body is at a 90 degree angle, with hands flat on the wall and your torso parallel to the floor. Keep your arms straight with a soft elbow so that your elbows are not locked.
- Slowly lift your left leg on your exhalation and feel a gentle lift in your core, as though you are supporting your baby from the inside out (see figure).
- Keep the standing leg straight and strong, and square your hips with the floor.
- Change sides.

Adjustments

If you have diastasis recti or if you are carrying multiples, omit this pose from your sequence.

Donkey Kick

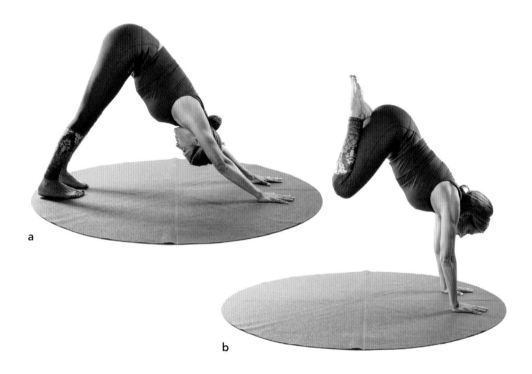

a

b

Benefits

This exercise strengthens the entire body, with emphasis on the triceps, the lower back, and the glutes.

Feeling

The feeling in the Donkey Kick is that of lifting the lower body as a preparation for eventually learning to jump to a handstand. Rather than focus on any specific pose as the goal, enjoy the feeling of having a little bit of hang time in the air. Stay playful and light with your attitude and your body.

Instruction

▋ Begin on your hands and knees with your hands shoulder width apart and your knees hip width apart.

▋ Lift your hips into Down Dog (see figure a).

▋ On your exhalation, kick your heels as though you were trying to kick your own bottom (see figure b). When your feet land on the ground, make sure to bend your knees to take any pressure off your lower back.

▋ Repeat as desired.

Adjustments

You can make this exercise easier by making the jump very small, just a few inches off of the floor.

Chair Pose Into Boat Pose

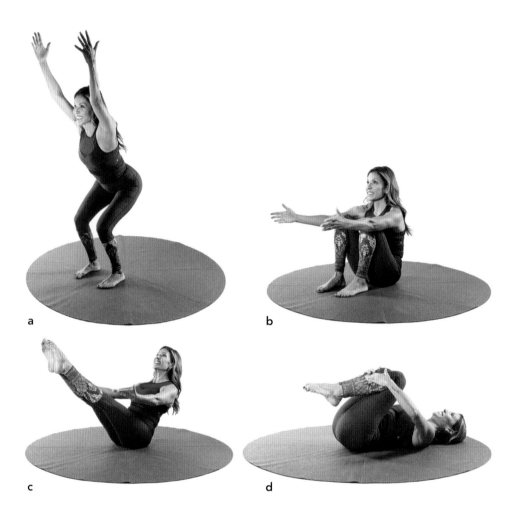

a

b

c

d

Benefits

This is a total body exercise, working several muscles as you move from standing to the floor and back up.

Feeling

Utkatasana, or Chair Pose, is also known as Lightning Bolt Pose, because it engenders a feeling of almost electric power. Feel that fiery energy when you are standing. In the transition to Boat Pose, the energy becomes that of water, or floating. This exercise offers the feeling of balance between fire and water, or yin and yang. Feel the power in your ability to move back and forth from being fierce to going with the flow. This is an important skill for moms; we protect our children fiercely, but we also go with the flow as we shed the illusion of control.

Instruction

- Begin standing with your feet hip width apart and your core muscles engaged.
- Lower your hips into a squat as though you were sitting in a chair. Make sure that your feet and your knees are the same distance apart, and that your knees are pointed straight forward (not bowing out or knocking in).
- Lift your arms overhead, working toward having your arms parallel with your ears (see figure a).
- Breathe deeply as you feel the strength in your quads and your core and sit deep into your squat until you can sit on the floor (see figure b).
- Once on the floor, lean your upper body back to a 45 degree angle and lift your legs to a 45 degree angle, with your feet together. Reach your arms straight in front of you and lift your breastbone into Boat Pose (see figure c).
- Maintain boat for 3-5 breaths, keeping your core muscles active.
- To transition back to Chair Pose from Boat Pose, lie down on your back and gently hug your knees to your chest (see figure d). Rock yourself forward to plant your feet onto the floor hip width apart, and return to standing.

Adjustments

If your shoulders are sensitive or tight, you can bring your arms into Cactus Pose while you are in Chair Pose. Cactus simply refers to bending the elbows so that your arms look like a goalpost. After you sit down, you can modify Boat Pose by bending your knees; this way there is less of a challenge for the abdomen. Choose this variation if you have lower back sensitivity.

Bow Pose

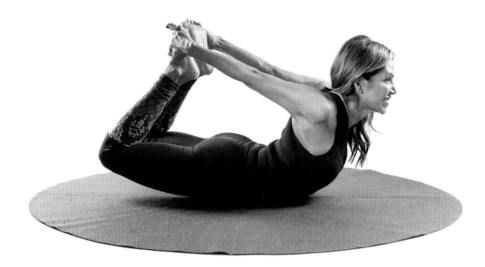

Benefits

This pose strengthens the muscles in the lower back. It also stretches the front of the body, including the abs, the chest, and the front of the shoulder.

Feeling

The name of the pose indicates the shape and the feeling, which are like an archer's bow and arrow. Where are you directing the arrow of your energy today? Before you move into Bow Pose, try closing your eyes and visualize an archer's bow. When you are ready, flutter your eyes open and create the shape with your body that you just envisioned.

Instruction

- Begin lying down on your abdomen with your feet no wider than hip width apart.
- Bend your knees and bring your hands to the corresponding top arch of the foot (right hand to right foot, left hand to left foot).
- Feel as though your feet are kicking back into your hands as you lift your chest and gently draw your shoulder blades in toward your spine.
- Breathe deeply and lift the thighs and chest off the floor (see figure).

Adjustments

To make this posture a bit easier, you can use a strap. Place the strap in your hands, and wrap it around the top arches of your feet. Lift the upper and lower body simultaneously.

Modified Side Plank Pose

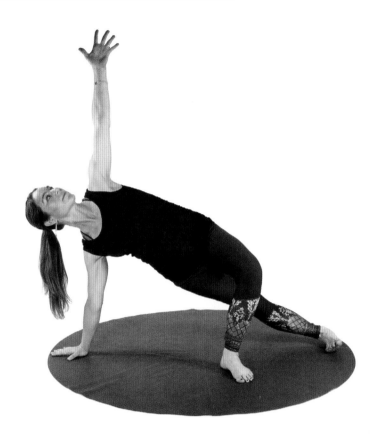

Benefit

This pose strengthens the stabilizers of the shoulder, triceps, and obliques.

Feeling

This variation of Full Side Plank has a similar feeling of supporting your body weight with the bottom arm. This movement requires strength and staying fully present in your body. Breathe into your sense of strength and power.

Instruction

- From Plank Pose (top of a push-up), place your right hand directly under your face and reach your left hand up to the sky.
- Step your left foot in front of you with the sole of your foot flat and your knee bent.
- Actively lift your hips and breathe deeply (see figure).
- Change sides.

Adjustments

If this exercise is very easy for you, you can stack or stagger your feet. The modification is great for pregnancy because the added weight of your beautiful baby belly is probably pulling your body forward. Modifying the exercise with the foot on the floor will make the exercise more accessible and easier to balance.

90-90 Stretch

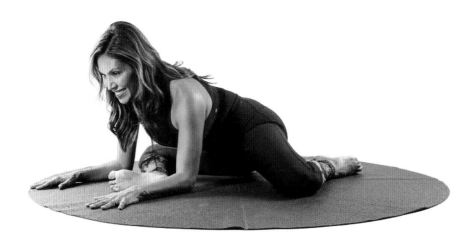

Benefits

This pose stretches the outer hip and thigh of the front leg as well as the quads and psoas of the back leg.

Feeling

As the name suggests, this stretch is very angular. Embrace this as a new way to stretch your body after pregnancy (which integrates more arcs and wavelike movements).

Instruction

- Begin seated on the floor with your legs extended in front of you.
- Turn your right knee to the right as you bend the knee to a 90 degree angle. Rotate the right hip outward.
- Draw your left leg behind you and bend your left knee to a 90 degree angle, with the left knee turned out to the left. You can keep the hands on the floor in front of you.
- Breathe slowly and deeply and maintain the stretch for at least 30 seconds. Change sides.

Adjustments

If you choose to deepen the stretch, place your elbows on the floor and easily fold forward to the extent that it feels good to stretch.

Putting It All Together

Included here are two practices aimed toward mamas in their 40s or older. The Independent Woman practice is a prenatal routine to help you ensure that there is balance in your body, specifically balance between the right and left sides, the upper and lower body, and the front and back of the body. The Jump for Joy practice is a postnatal routine designed to give you a jumpstart—literally and figuratively—to reclaiming your strength.

Society has a lot to say about women having babies in their 40s. Let go of the outside voices and hear your own confident voice guiding you in meditation; let that confidence inspire your movement today and every day. The name of this workout is a double entendre: In addition to being designed for an independent, confident woman, it focuses on bilateral movement, which simply means one side working independently of the other. It's normal to favor your dominant side. If you're right-handed you might favor your right side, or if this isn't your first pregnancy you might have another child on your left hip or shoulder much of the time to leave your right hand free to open a car door or answer a phone call, for example. This workout will expose any imbalances you might have between right and left, and allow you the opportunity to cultivate balance and let the two sides strengthen independently. You can enjoy this routine two or three days a week, along with walking for at least 20 to 30 minutes on the alternate days. As always, check with your doctor before beginning this or any other exercise program.

Exercise	Page	Focus	Reps/Time
Meditation in Mountain Pose	45	Centering energy	9 slow, deep, centering breaths, focusing on the inhalation and the exhalation being equal in length
Half Sun Salutation	48	Shoulders, core strength, flexibility	3 rounds; remember that each movement corresponds to an inhalation or exhalation
Firedancer Squat	258	Lower body focus, especially the glutes, quads, deep core muscles, pelvic floor muscles	2-3 sets of 10 reps
Alternating Reverse Lunge	241	Lower body	2-3 sets of 10-12 reps on the right and left

> continued

Independent Woman   *> continued*

Exercise	Page	Focus	Reps/Time
Standing Hip Abduction	90	Outer thighs and hips	2 sets of 12-15 reps
Running Man	261	TVA, shoulders	2 sets of 20 reps total using 3-5 lb weights
Modified Side Plank Pose	267	Obliques, triceps	3-5 deep breaths with the right hand on the floor and then 3-5 deep breaths with the left hand on the floor; option to repeat both sides
Warrior 3 Pose With Hands on Wall	262	Stabilizers of the standing leg, hamstring of the lifted leg, core strength	5 deep breaths on each side; option to repeat on both sides
Pigeon Pose	56	Outer hips, lower back	9 deep breaths on each side
IT Band Twist	57	IT band	5 deep breaths right and left
Fish Pose	196	Pecs, abs	5 deep breaths with a block or bolster under midback
Deep Relaxation Pose	66	Entire body	1-3 minutes

Whether you had a baby 8 weeks ago or 18 years ago, getting in shape over the age of 40 is a little bit different than getting in shape at the age of 20. As we get older, our metabolism slows down and it is necessary to give the body a bit more of a challenge to jumpstart the metabolism. This practice incorporates plyometric training to get you jumping for joy! If you find that you have light bladder leakage (LBL) when jumping, try doing a Kegel at the top of each jump. Not only will this help with LBL, it is what the yogis call *mula bandha*, which means *root lock*, as discussed earlier. Root lock refers to the muscles of the pelvic floor. By lifting the pelvic floor, you will have a lighter landing with more power. This should be practiced on the landing phase of each jump in plyometrics. Note: Shoes are optional for this workout. If you decide to wear shoes, be sure they have adequate cushioning (i.e., they are less than one year old).

Exercise	Page	Focus	Reps/Time
Garland Pose	63	Centering energy	9 slow, deep, centering breaths focusing on the inhalation and the exhalation being equal in length
Squat	257	Lower body and core stabilizers	3 sets of 10-12 reps
Squat Jump	259	Entire body, with emphasis on lower body and core	3 sets of 10-12 reps
Burpee	240	Entire body	3 sets of 5-8 reps

> continued

Jump for Joy *> continued*

Exercise	Page	Focus	Reps/Time
Jumping Lunge	260	Entire body, with emphasis on lower body and core	3 sets of 10-12 reps (total)
Donkey Kick	263	Entire body, with emphasis on lower body and core	3 sets of 10-12 reps (total)
Chair Pose Into Boat Pose	264	Entire body, with emphasis on lower body and core	3 sets of 8-10 reps
90-90 Stretch	268	Outer hip of the front leg, quads and psoas of the back leg	9 deep breaths on the right and left sides
Boat Pose Into Bridge Pose	264, 155	Lower back, TVA, abs	10 reps of each pose, performed at a slow, smooth pace
Seated Twist	217	Core stabilizers (stretching)	5 deep breaths right, 5 deep breaths left
Bow Pose	266	Lower back, abdomen, front of the shoulders	5 deep breaths
Garland Pose	63	Centering energy	9 slow, deep, centering breaths. focusing on the inhalation and the exhalation being equal in length

Speaking Your Truth

When you are pregnant, other people naturally want to connect with the miracle that you are experiencing. Very often complete strangers will walk up to you and start telling you terrible stories about their own or their best friend's pregnancy. Some people may start touching your belly when your beautiful baby bump is showing. I can't imagine doing any of this. Everyone is different, though, and my views on people's unwanted remarks and touch have softened with age. I choose to believe that people often make these errors innocently in an effort to connect with something wonderful. They see the beauty of your pregnancy and want to touch it. Or they see that beautiful belly and assume that it is uncomfortable and want to commiserate. In these situations, as always, it's OK to speak your truth.

Speaking your truth is not always easy, and sometimes we have to feel the fear and do it anyway. If someone is touching your belly and you prefer that they do not, it's OK to gently move their hand away and say, "I prefer that you do not touch my belly." If it is someone in your family and you are concerned with what they might think of you, I encourage you to remember that it is up to you to set boundaries. Setting healthy boundaries during pregnancy makes it much easier to set healthy boundaries after your baby is born.

As I get older, I find that confidence and boldness also come with age. More and more women are having babies in their 40s and while some might argue that it is harder to have a baby at a later age, I can tell you firsthand that there are advantages as well. One of the advantages that I experienced in my pregnancy is that it gave me the courage to speak up for myself. Like many young women, I used to suffer from the need to please others and have them like me. I remember attending a yoga class with a high-profile yoga teacher when I was pregnant with my first child. This teacher had the whole class move into a Standing Twist. He called me out in front of the class, asking "Are you injured?" I reminded him that I was pregnant, and he said, "My wife did that pose while she was pregnant and she was fine." I should have walked out of the class at that moment, but I wanted him to like me as a colleague.

During the second trimester of my second pregnancy, in my 40s, I once found myself in a similar situation. This time I was in a different teacher's class and he suggested that I move into Cobra on my belly. I said, "You want me to lie on my baby?" I scared the heck out of him and made myself smile at my newfound confidence in speaking my truth.

I am not suggesting that it is necessary to call people out when they give bad information, but you also don't have to listen. By the time we're in our 40s, most of us have learned who we are and what makes us tick. If something doesn't resonate with you, if someone is trying to scare you, intimidate you, or give you poor information, it's OK to walk away. And yes, that goes for yoga teachers and personal trainers too. Your inner wisdom will guide you and your body will let you know if something feels right or not. Listen to your body's wisdom and trust your internal processes.

*M*ommy Move

Active Bridges

Bridge Pose in yoga focuses a little bit more on the lower back than on the glutes. Bridge in fitness focuses a lot on the glutes. I have practiced the pose both ways and find that it is the exact same movement, but you can choose what part of the body you would like to emphasize by putting your attention on that particular body part. For me, I love glute bridges, and am a bit of a rebel in the yoga community when I say "Flex your glutes" at the top of Bridge Pose. As a mom, I know the benefits of posterior chain training and any movement that targets the posterior chain is great work. I like to blend the two systems of movement. Here is how I cue active glute bridges.

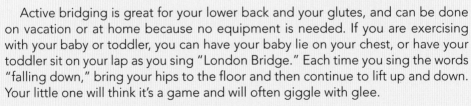

▌ Begin lying down on your back with your knees bent and your feet hip width apart. Make sure that all your toes are pointed straight forward and that your knees are directly over your ankles (see figure a).

▌ Slowly lift your hips as high as you comfortably can while you easily create a sense of expansion across your chest and of length in your abdomen (see figure b). You can choose to hold onto the sides of the yoga mat if you have tight shoulders, or you can keep your hands flat on the floor if your shoulders are a little more open.

▌ Keeping all the toes pointed forward at the top of the movement, contract your glutes and allow this powerful muscle group to assist the lift. Feel a sense of spaciousness in the heart center, and breathe.

▌ Now lower and lift your hips for 10 reps, contracting the glutes each time you lift.

Active bridging is great for your lower back and your glutes, and can be done on vacation or at home because no equipment is needed. If you are exercising with your baby or toddler, you can have your baby lie on your chest, or have your toddler sit on your lap as you sing "London Bridge." Each time you sing the words "falling down," bring your hips to the floor and then continue to lift up and down. Your little one will think it's a game and will often giggle with glee.

Information No One Tells You

PMS and Caffeine

For women all over the world, premenstrual syndrome can bring mood swings, weight fluctuations, headaches, bloating, and other unpleasant manifestations. Researchers have found that caffeine consumption can increase the severity of PMS. At the other end of the spectrum, there is research demonstrating that there are moderate health benefits from caffeine. For Mothers Into Living Fit, I recommend being somewhere in the middle, reducing caffeine consumption but not necessarily cutting it out altogether. Try limiting your consumption to 200 to 300 mg daily, which is the equivalent of a tall cup of coffee. Also, be aware that there is caffeine in more than just coffee. Some sources of caffeine that might be hiding in your diet include soda, chocolate, ice cream, and of course, energy drinks.

Love-Your-Baby Visualization

Scanning Your Body's Story

Lying down in Relaxation Pose, spread out and get comfortable. If you have an eye pillow, you might want to cover your eyes so you can turn your attention inward on a slightly deeper level and withdraw your senses from outside stimuli. The yogis call this *pratyahara*, meaning *sense withdrawal*. Slow your breath down and easily sense your thoughts slowing down too. Allow your focus and attention to move to the left side of your body. Breathe into the left lung, and into the left side waist. Now slowly scan your body on the left side (only) from your left foot all the way up to the left side of your head. Notice any tattoos, scars, injuries, traumas, and joys that occurred on this side of your body. What is the story of this side? What memories come up when you connect to the left side of your body? Are there any labels or judgments that you associate with this side of your body? Is it the strong side? Is it the flexible side? Does this side of your body hold any stories that that no longer serve you? Breathe deeply and feel your deep breath easily detaching you from the pain of the past. Try to see yourself as the heroine of any challenging situations, because in fact you are. You are here, now, and you have survived all previous traumas and challenges. Send light, love, and positive energy to this entire side of your body.

Now slowly allow your focus and attention to drift to the right side of your body and once again scan this side of your body from your right foot, all the way up to the right side of your head. Notice any stories, feelings, thoughts, and memories associated with this side of your body. Breathe into this side of your body and once again, send light, love, and positive energy to every part of the right side of your body.

> continued

Easily allow your attention to drift to the midline of your body, to your spine, what the yogis call the tree of life. Allow both sides of your body to unite harmoniously at this center line. If any trauma or struggle has occurred at the midline of your body, feel the two sides of your body supporting and strengthening your midline. Envision your body as luminous and joyous from your feet all the way up to the top of your head and beyond. Slowly allow your attention to drift back to the present, to this moment, and breathe into your strength. Remember that you are the heroine of your own story. Thank your body for all that it has done for you and continues to do for you. *Shanti.* Peace

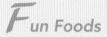# Fun Foods

Dark Chocolate

Dark chocolate is readily available in many stores and has many health benefits. Here are some of the health benefits of dark chocolate:

- Potential for cancer prevention
- Antioxidant-rich superfood
- Potential for improved heart health
- Improved brain function
- Blood pressure aid
- Rich in antioxidants

When purchasing dark chocolate, look for fair trade or organic chocolate with 70 percent or higher total cocoa content, where sugar is listed as the last ingredient and there are no trans fats. Choose a brand with a taste that fits your palate (it should be yummy) and try to stick with no more than one ounce of dark chocolate daily.

Bibliography

American College of Obstetricians and Gynecologists (ACOG). July 2017. "Frequently Asked Questions Pregnancy." https://www.acog.org/Patients/FAQs/Exercise-During-Pregnancy

American College of Sports Medicine (ACSM). "The ACSM Definition of Cardiovascular Exercise." https://livehealthy.chron.com/acsm-definition-cardiovascular-exercise-7996.html

American College of Sports Medicine (ACSM). "Resistance Training For Health And Fitness." https://www.prescriptiontogetactive.com/app/uploads/resistance-training-ACSM.pdf

Babycenter. 2018. "Your Six-Week Postpartum Checkup." www.babycenter.com/0_your-six-week-postpartum-checkup_1152300.bc

Better Movement. "The SAID Principle." www.bettermovement.org/blog/2009/0110111

Carney, D.R., A.J.C. Cuddy, and A.J. Yap. 2010. "Power Posing: Brief Nonverbal Displays Affect NeuroendocrineLevels and Risk Tolerance." http://datacolada.org/wp-content/uploads/2015/05/Carney-Cuddy-Yap-2010.pdf

Centers for Disease Control (CDC). "Healthy Pregnant or Postpartum Women." https://www.cdc.gov/physicalactivity/basics/pregnancy/index.htm

Centers for Disease Control (CDC). 2018. "Physical Activity Guidelines." www.cdc.gov/cancer/dcpc/prevention/policies_practices/physical_activity/guidelines.htm

Chopra, D. "5 Steps to Harness the Power of Intention." www.mindbodygreen.com/0-9603/5-steps-to-harness-the-power-of-intention.html

Chopra, D. 2005. *Magical Beginnings, Enchanted Lives*. New York: Three Rivers Press.

Clapp, J. 2012. *Exercising Through Your Pregnancy*. Omaha, NE: Addicus Books.

Cornish, J.L. Personal interview.

Crawford, N. "Exercising With Your Baby: The Babywearing Workout." https://breakingmuscle.com/fitness/exercising-with-your-baby-the-babywearing-workout

Csikszentmihalyi, M.

Fit For Birth. N.D. "A Mother's Emotions Affect Her Unborn Child." http://getfitforbirth.com/a-mothers-emotions-affect-her-unborn-child

Gaskin, I.M. "Reducing Fear of Birth in U.S. Culture." https://www.youtube.com/watch?v=S9LO1Vb54yk

Guha, A. 2006. "Ayurvedic Concept of Food and Nutrition." http://opencommons.uconn.edu/cgi/viewcontent.cgi?article=1025&context=som_articles

Livestrong. "13 Benefits of Weightlifting That No One Tells You About." www.livestrong.com/slideshow/1008208-13-benefits-weightlifting-one-tells

Mayo Clinic. "Healthy Pregnant or Postpartum Women." https://www.cdc.gov/physicalactivity/basics/pregnancy/index.htm

Merriam-Webster. www.merriam-webster.com/dictionary/intention

Michael, R. "What Self-Care Is—and What It Isn't." *Psych Central*. https://psychcentral.com/blog/what-self-care-is-and-what-it-isnt-2

Morin, A. "The Secret of Becoming Mentally Strong." https://www.youtube.com/watch?v=T-Fbv757kup4

National Fitness Hall of Fame. 2007. www.nationalfitnesshalloffame.com/sattlerdrthomas.html

Orloff, J. 2014. "Yahoo Parenting: Is A 'Mother's Intuition' Real?" https://drjudithorloff.com/is-mothers-intuition-real/

Rosen, R. 2014. "Who Was Patanjali?" *Yoga Journal.* www.yogajournal.com/yoga-101/who-was-patanjali

Sattler, Thomas. Personal interview.

Wikipedia. "Linea Alba (Abdomen)." https://en.wikipedia.org/wiki/Linea_alba_(abdomen)

Wikipedia. "Linea nigra." https://en.wikipedia.org/wiki/Linea_nigra

Wilkes, C., M. Sagar, R.R. Kidd, and E. Broadbent. 2017. "Upright Posture Improves Affect and Fatigue in People With Depressive Symptoms." www.researchgate.net/publication/305760982_Upright_posture_improves_affect_and_fatigue_in_people_with_depressive_symptoms

Wilson, J. 2017. "How Much Is Too Much Exercise When You're Pregnant?" www.cnn.com/2013/09/20/health/pregnant-woman-weightlifter-crossfit/index.html

About the Author

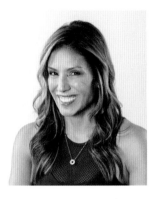

Desi Bartlett MS, CPT E-RYT, has been teaching health and wellness for over 20 years. She is a dynamic motivator and widely sought after international presenter and spokesperson. Her teaching approach taps into one's inner joy and makes movement an outer expression of that state.

Originally from Chicago, Bartlett earned a degree in kinesiology, with a minor in dance, and a master's degree in corporate fitness. She holds advanced certifications in yoga, personal training, pre- and postnatal fitness, and group fitness. She is a continuing education provider through the National Academy of Sports Medicine and the National Council for Certified Personal Trainers. She has worked with the U.S. Navy and with several large companies, including Manduka, Gaiam, Equinox, and Mattel.

Bartlett has worked with several celebrity moms in Los Angeles, including Alicia Silverstone and Kate Hudson. Her inspiring and unique classes have been featured on networks such as ABC, NBC, FOX, Univision, Hallmark, and Lifetime. She is passionate about communicating her message of the joy of movement with people all over the world, and her DVDs are distributed in the United States, Latin America, and Europe. She currently stars in eight yoga, fitness, and dance DVDs, including *Better Belly Yoga*, *Latin Groove*, and *Total Body Tone*. She has a diverse background in many areas of fitness and yoga and has worked as a product director for Gaiam and as the group fitness manager for Equinox Santa Monica, and she created a new round yoga mat for Manduka. She is currently a Manduka ambassador and their director of community events.

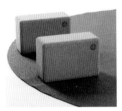
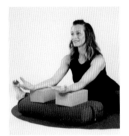
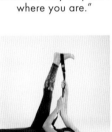
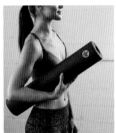
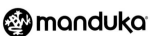

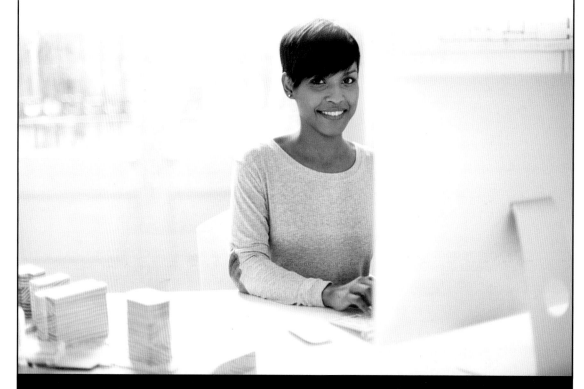
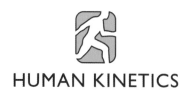